Fighting For This Life
Our Cancer Journey

Justin Bowen & Helga Peeters

Independently Published

ISBN 978-1-9168746-0-2 (Paperback)
ISBN 978-1-9168746-1-9 (epub)
First printing edition 2021

With much appreciation for
Book Design: Alison Keys Creative
Advice and Guidance: Alison Jean Lester and Andy Gurnett

For

Bren and Seren

with love always...

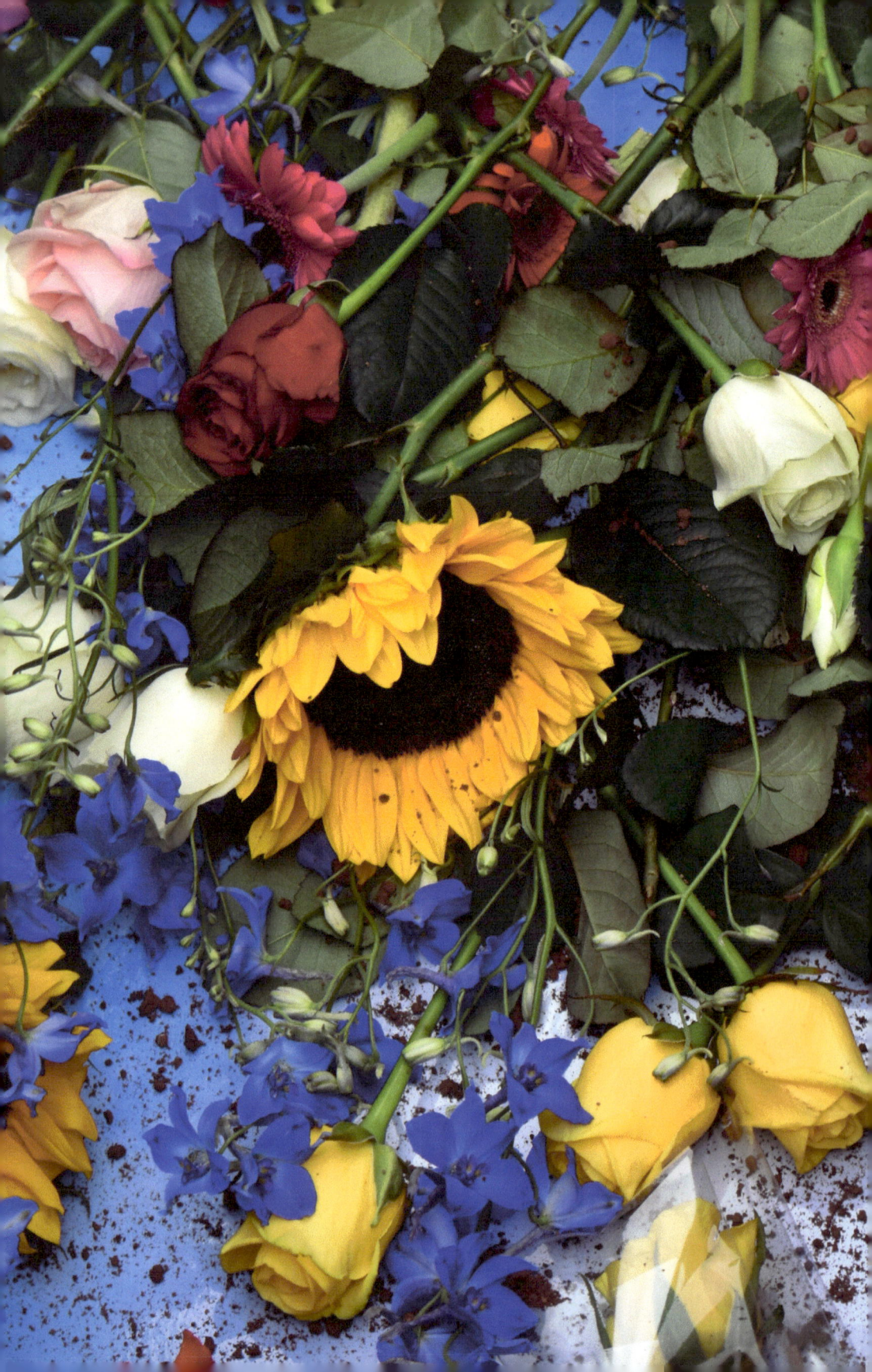

Introduction

When my wife Helga was diagnosed with breast cancer in June 2016, we began a journey of indeterminate length, unimaginable twists and an unknown destination.

We knew that at some point it was likely to end in Helga's death, but in truth there was a spectrum of possibilities that spanned our worst nightmares to our most wishful dreams.

So, after the initial shock and grief of that first diagnosis, we resolved to live our lives as if every moment could be Helga's last, but with the unshakeable belief that she could also live a long and happy life.

We also knew that we would need the support of all of our family and friends.

Now Helga was one of those people who seemed to know, and get along with, everyone. In addition, being from Belgium and working in a multinational company, her network spanned many different countries and so keeping everyone informed was going to be a challenge.

So we decided to make full use of that most remarkable of modern inventions, social media - and we decided to use the biggest platform of them all...

Facebook.
Justin Bowen - September 2020

Justin Bowen
15th Jun 2016 at 11:57

As some of you know, Helga was diagnosed with breast cancer a couple of weeks ago. Rather than have multiple conversations, we've decided to keep people updated here on Facebook as to how it's going.

The first thing to say is you'll not hear any moaning. Life is brutal, but it also brought us together and has given us 2 delightful children, so life is wonderful too. We appreciate what we have and won't complain about this. What we know so far is that Helga has 3 lumps inside her breast and the cancer is fast growing. However, it is of a type that is hormonal and so is susceptible to some very effective drugs - that is good news!

The cancer has also not spread beyond the breast, which is more good news! That was the thing we were most worried about, so when we heard this we decided it warranted a glass of wine by way of a celebration. We intend celebrating whenever we can, all the way until Helga is better.

Helga will have chemotherapy first to shrink the tumours. She'll have 6 to 8 treatments, with 3 weeks between each treatment. There will be side effects, such as nausea, tiredness, low immunity and hair loss. I've told Helga not to worry about the hair loss - I've had it for 20 years and have a perfectly good set of clippers she is welcome to use. Once the chemo treatments are finished, Helga will have surgery to remove one or both breasts.

This will be a long haul and we're under no illusions that it will be an almighty challenge. But we're lucky to have good family and friends so fully expect to come out the other side in good shape.

The children think it's hilarious that mummy is going to lose her hair. Seren just wanted another biscuit for supper. So, life goes on! We'll update as we go and see you all as and when we can!

Love Justin and Helga...

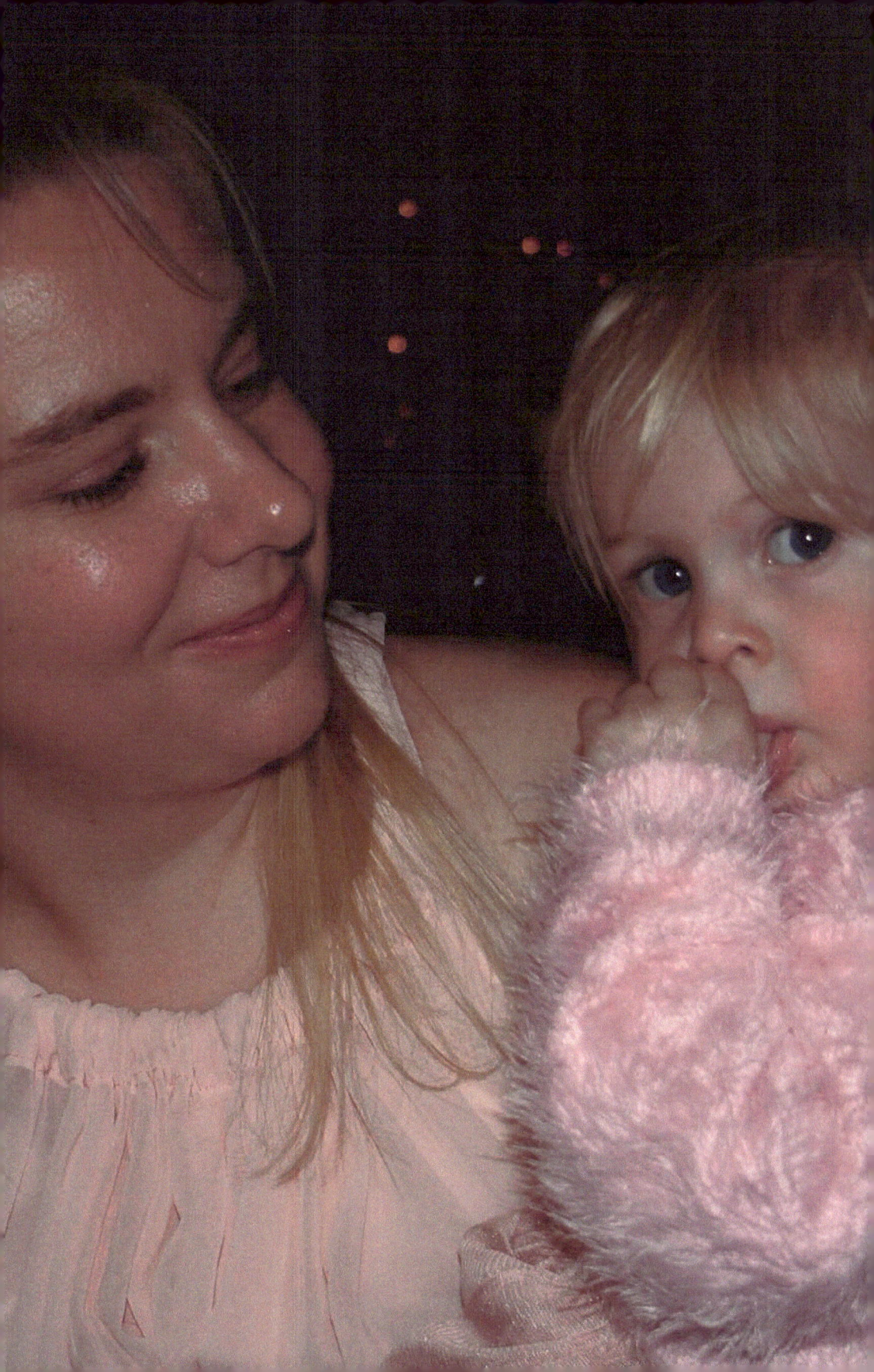

HELGA BEGAN HER FIRST COURSE OF
CHEMOTHERAPY THE FOLLOWING
WEEK. IT INVOLVED A COMBINATION OF
DRUGS CALLED FEC-TH WHICH WOULD
BE ADMINISTERED EVERY 3 WEEKS
INTRAVENOUSLY AT THE HOSPITAL. THE
FIRST NOTICEABLE EFFECT WAS THAT
HELGA'S HAIR STARTED TO FALL OUT.

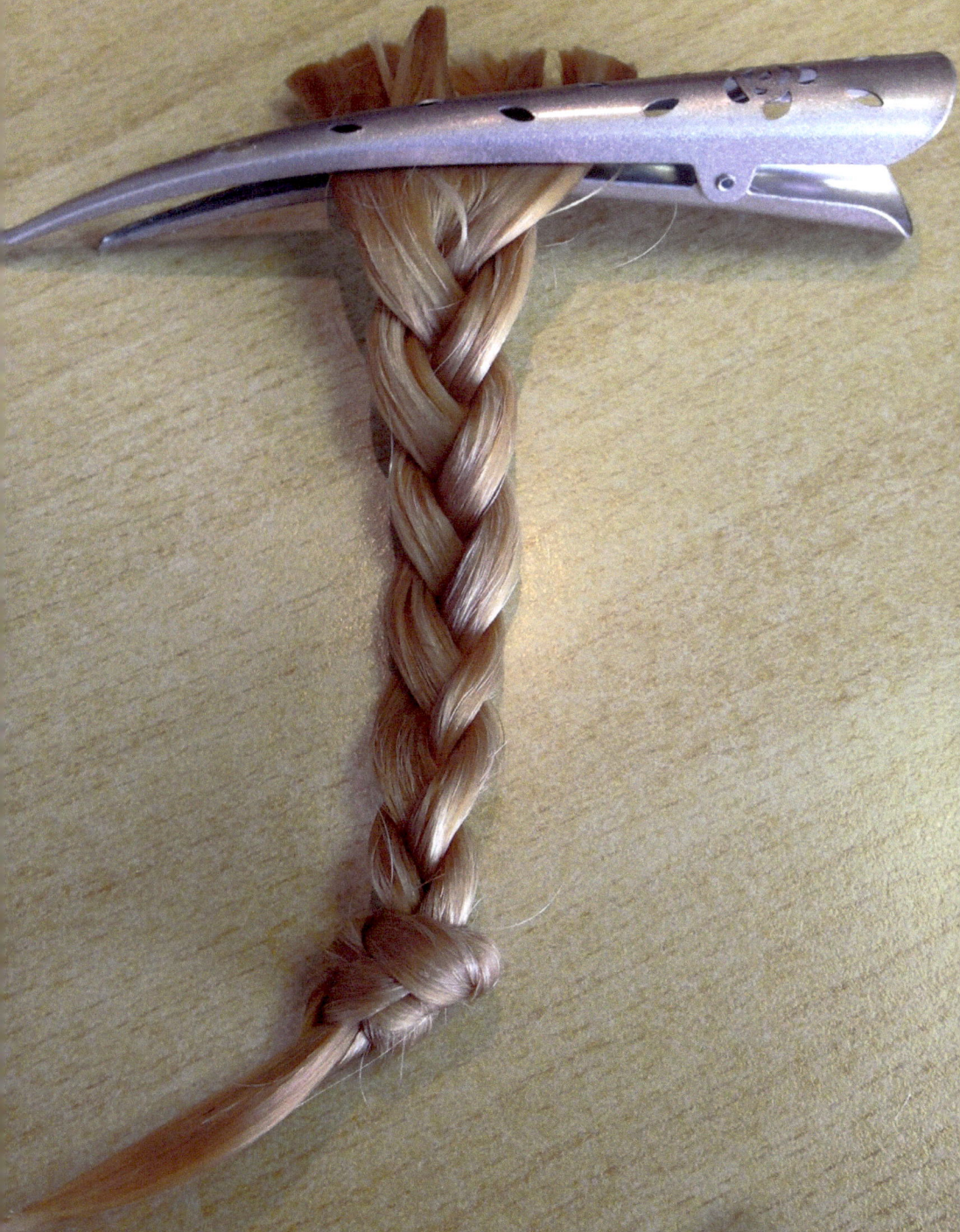

Justin Bowen
25th Jun 2016 at 15:01

Out trying wigs on with Mummy...

Helga Peeters is 😊 **feeling amused** with **Justin Bowen**
15th July 2016 at 09:40 · Droitwich

On the 9th wedding anniversary day my true love and kids gave meeeee...
A shave and a hat!

😂

Don't think I've ever been so quick in the morning with a towel dry of my head

👍

Happy anniversary darling!

🎉

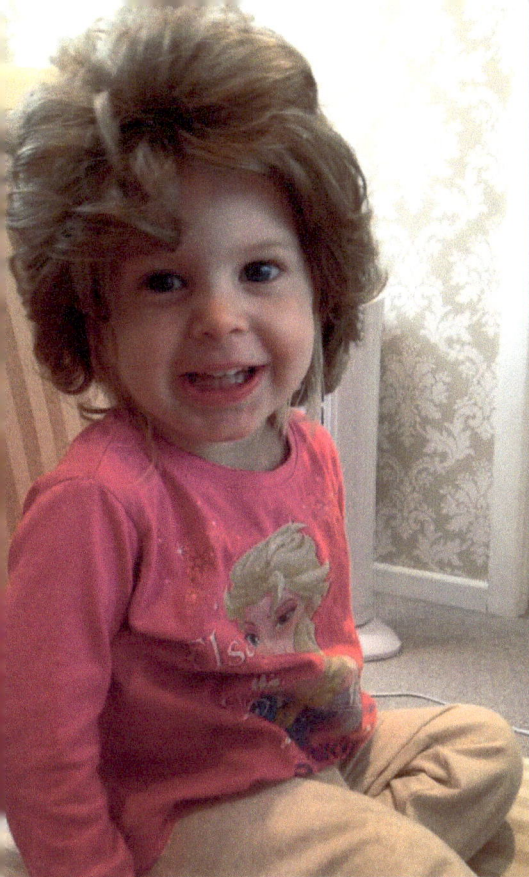

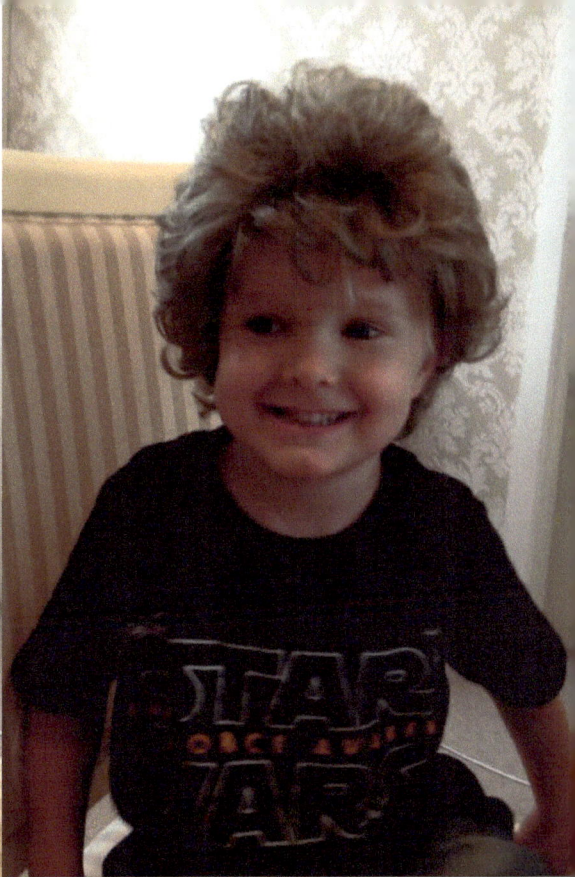

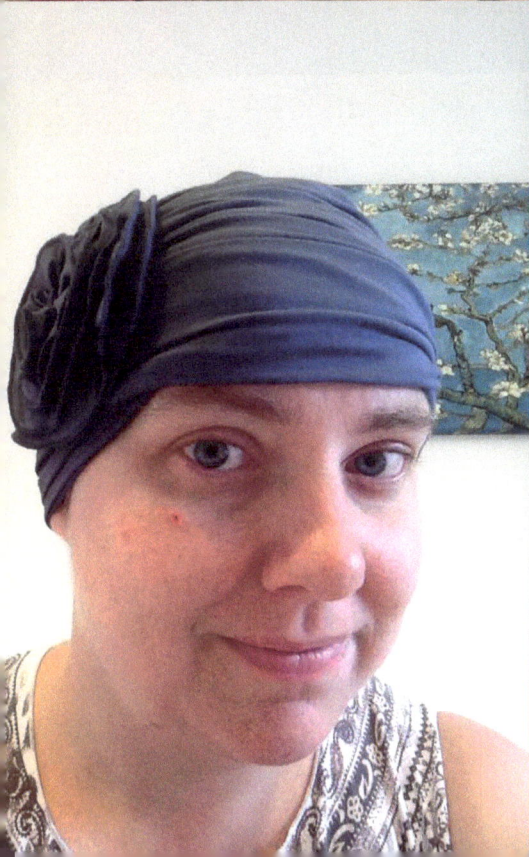

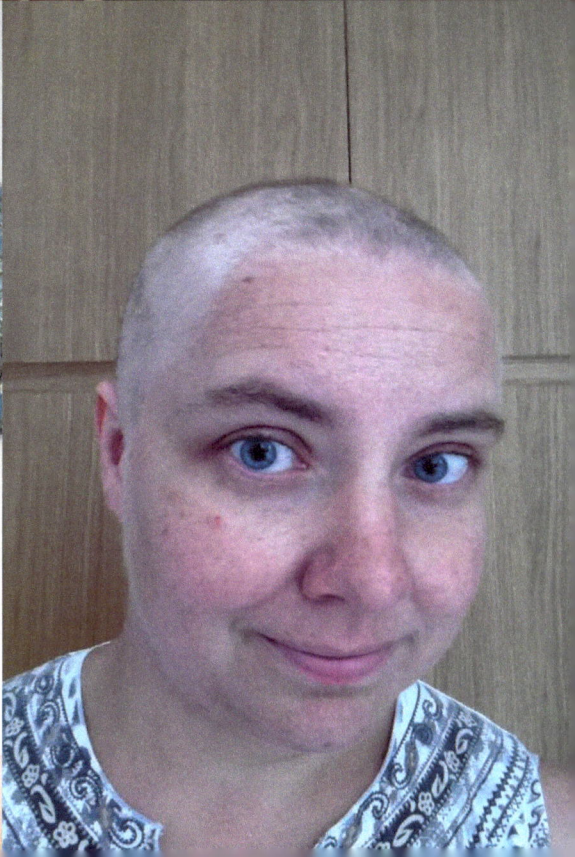

AFTER 2 ROUNDS OF CHEMOTHERAPY, HELGA
HAD A SCAN TO SEE IF THE TREATMENT WAS
PROVING EFFECTIVE AND SHRINKING
THE CANCER.

AN APPOINTMENT WAS MADE TO SEE HER
ONCOLOGIST ON 1ST AUGUST 2016, WHEN
WE WOULD GET THE RESULTS.

THE WAIT BETWEEN THE SCAN AND THE
RESULT IS ONE OF THE HARDEST TIMES
IN CANCER TREATMENT. HELGA CALLED
IT "SCANXIETY". EMOTIONS CAN SWING
BETWEEN WANTING TO KNOW, NOT
WANTING TO KNOW, HOPING FOR THE BEST,
FEARING THE WORST. YOU HAVE TO KEEP
PUTTING IT OUT OF YOUR MIND UNTIL THE
MOMENT COMES WHEN YOU ACTUALLY
HEAR THE RESULT...

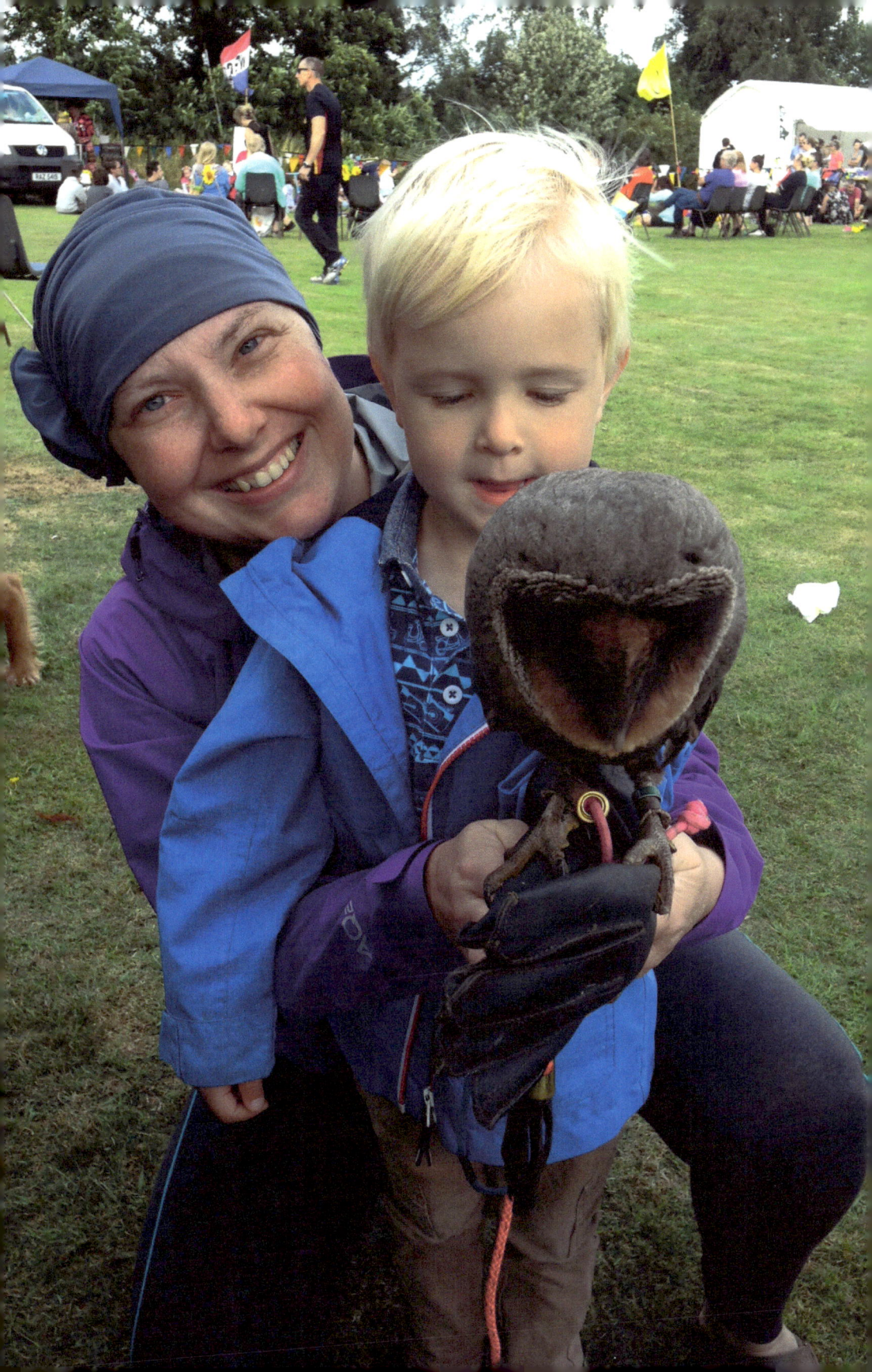

Justin Bowen
1st August 2016 at 20:11 · Droitwich

"Oh that's better!" said Helga's consultant today during her latest examination. Heading into the third cycle of treatment and that is EXACTLY the kind of line we wanted to hear. So this little beauty has been opened, by way of a small celebration, one step further along the road to good health.

Shiraz

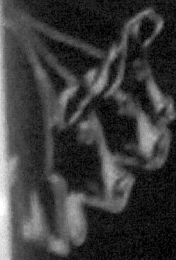

16 Little Black Pigs

South Eastern Australia

THE RESULT WAS A HUGE RELIEF. THE TUMOURS HAD SHRUNK SIGNIFICANTLY AND, FOR NOW AT LEAST, A HUGE WEIGHT HAD BEEN LIFTED FROM OUR SHOULDERS. IT GAVE US CONFIDENCE TO LOOK FORWARD WITH OPTIMISM AND STRENGTHENED OUR RESOLVE TO LIVE POSITIVELY. WE DECIDED A LITTLE HOLIDAY WAS IN ORDER.

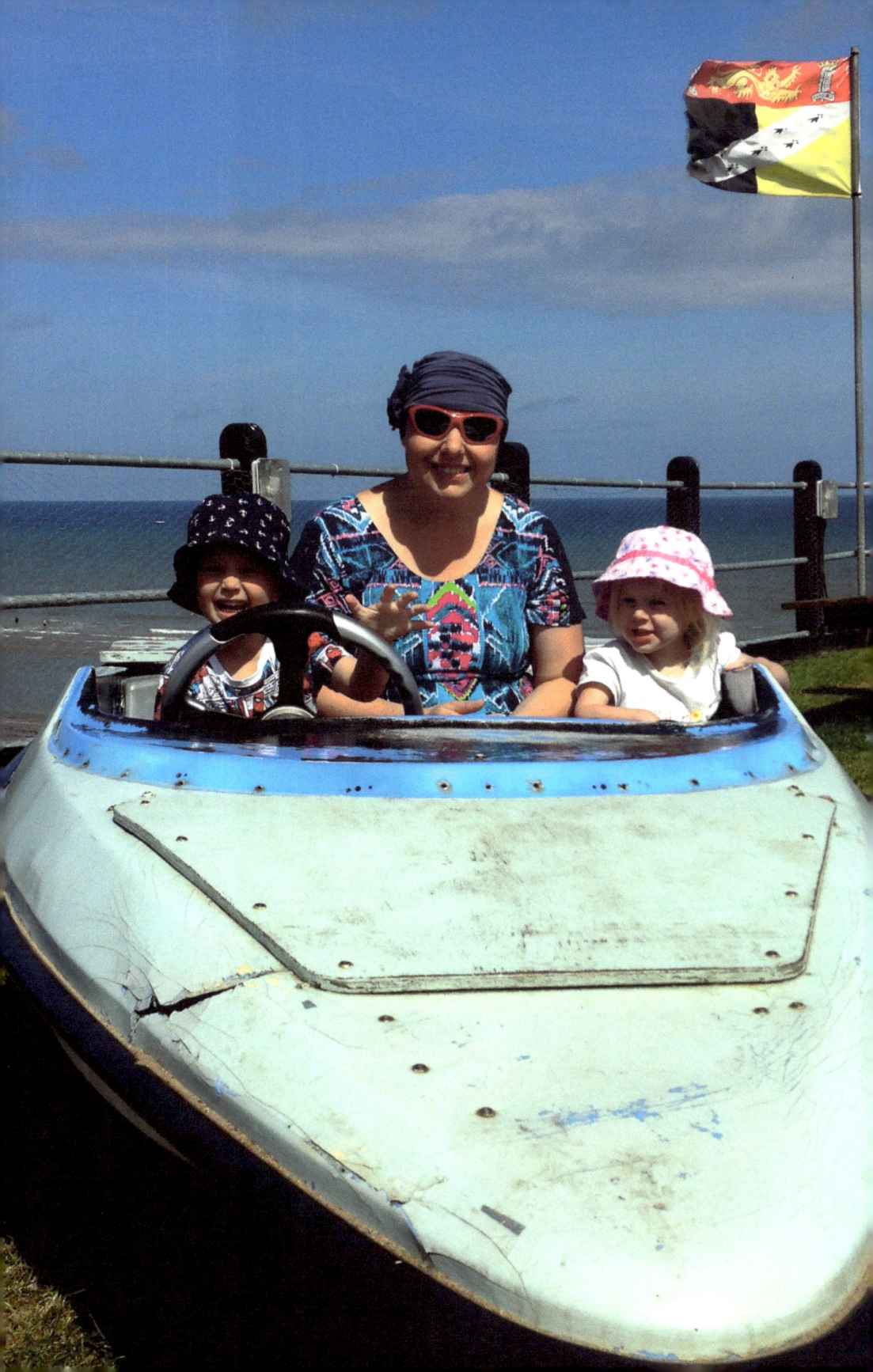

Justin Bowen is with **Helga Peeters** at **Mundesley Beach Front**
16th August 2016 at 14:53 · Norfolk

Fun on the Beach!

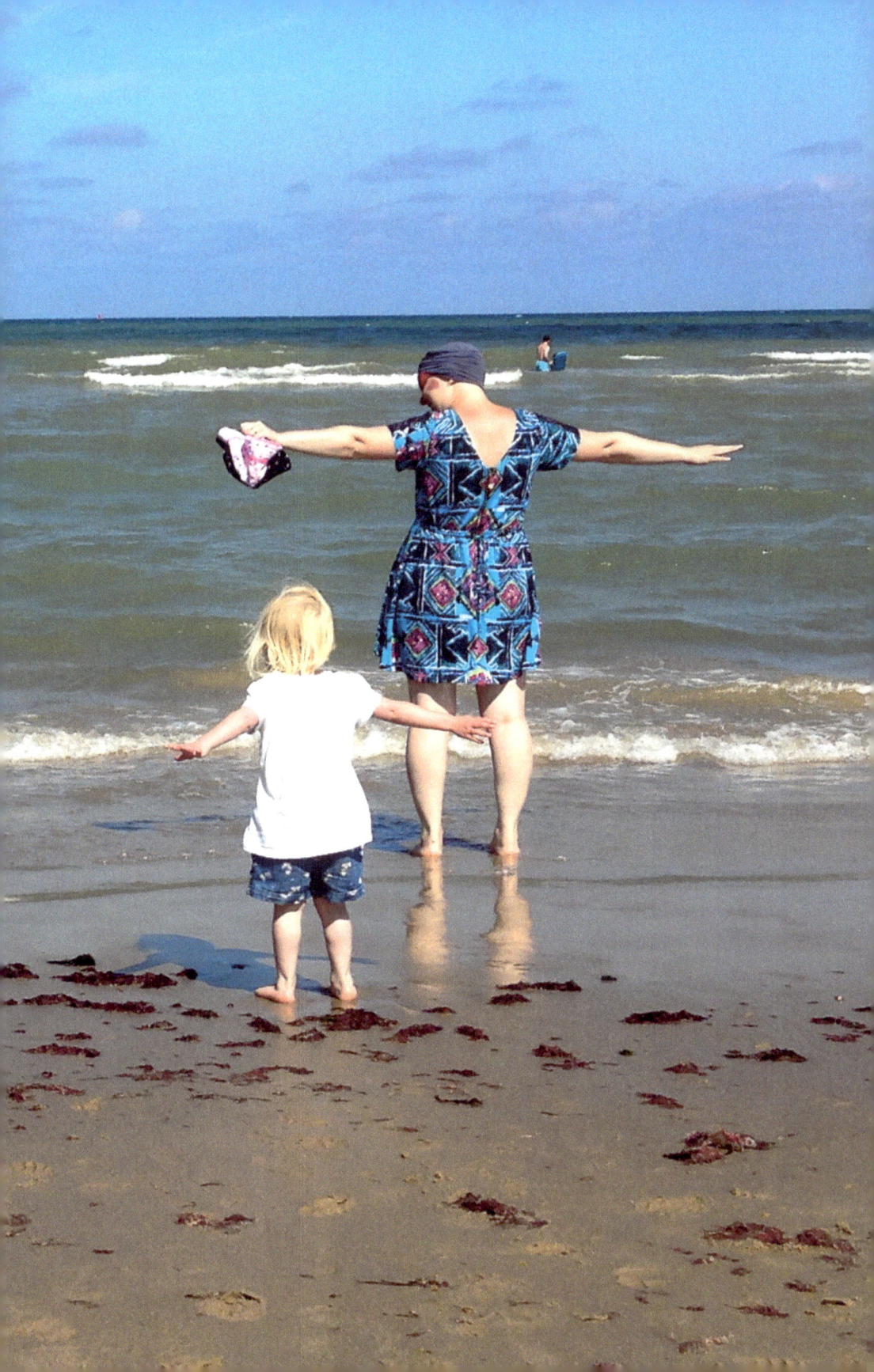

HELGA'S TREATMENT CONTINUED WITH
3-WEEKLY CYCLES. MEANWHILE, THE
GENETICS TEAM AT ADDENBROOKE'S
HOSPITAL CAMBRIDGE WERE LOOKING
AT WHETHER HELGA'S CANCER WAS
HEREDITARY, GIVEN THAT HELGA HAD A
LONG FAMILY HISTORY OF BREAST CANCER.
IT TURNED OUT THAT THERE WAS INDEED A
GENE THAT HAD CAUSED HER CANCER.

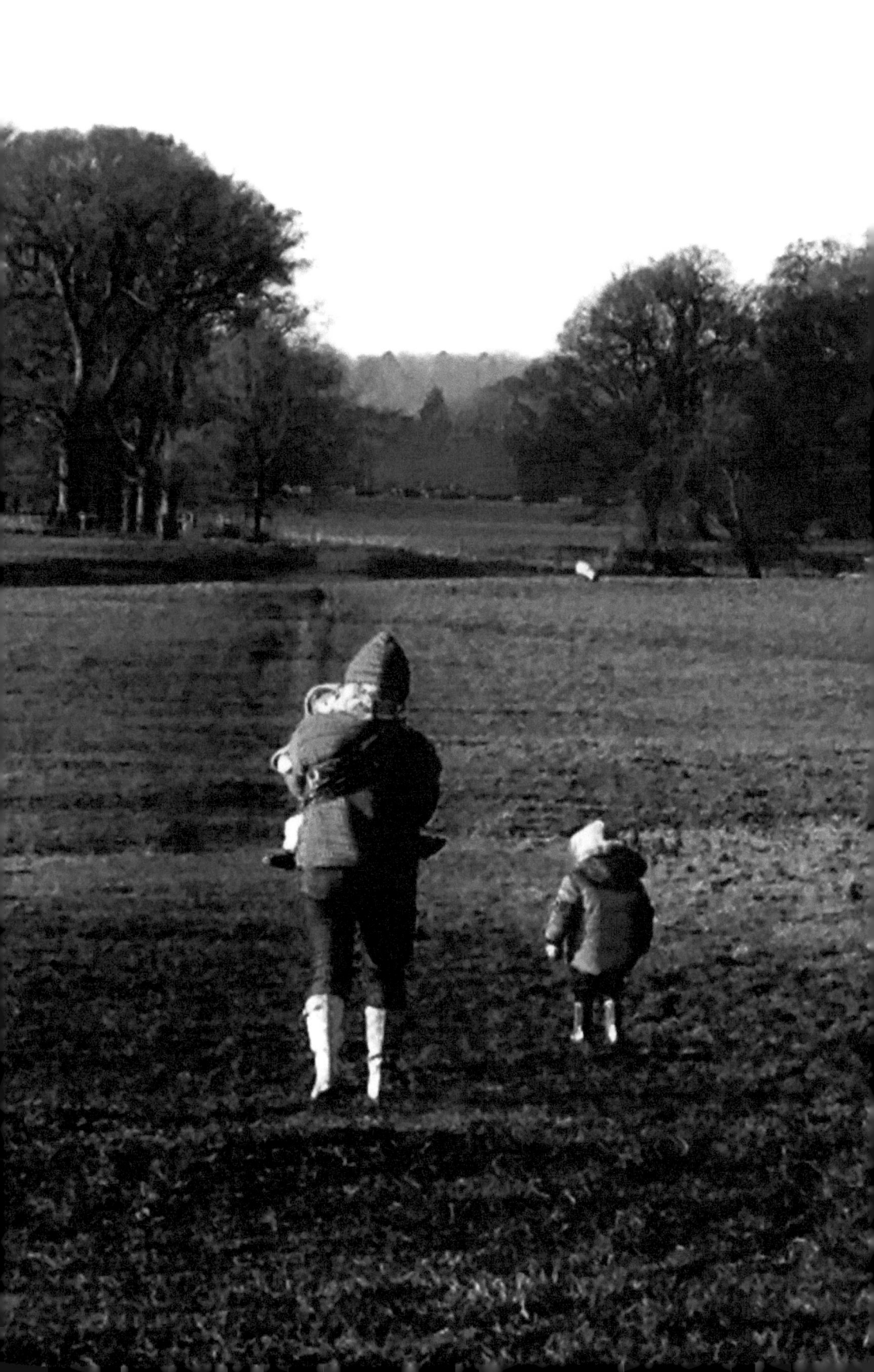

Justin Bowen updated his status
16th Sep 2016 at 19:58 · Droitwich

So we've had a fuller explanation now from the Worcester Genetics Team about the gene which has caused Helga's breast cancer.

It's the PalB2 gene and it has a 50% chance of being passed from mother to daughter when it's in an altered state. Not much is known about it, other than it causes breast cancer if it's mutated. So if you have the altered version of this gene and you're female you're likely to get breast cancer. Doesn't matter what you eat, drink, smoke, do - chances are you'll cop it. And then there's a 50% chance it will pass to your children.

Which all comes back to life being what it is. It has given us 2 wonderful kids. It's given Helga this mutated gene (I can't help but think X-Men when I hear that) and it might have passed onto our kids. It's given me short legs and a bald head, which they might also have been lucky enough to inherit.

Are we going to worry about this? F**k no. What we're going to do is go to Alton Towers on Sunday and have a lovely day. Then we'll carry on getting Helga better.

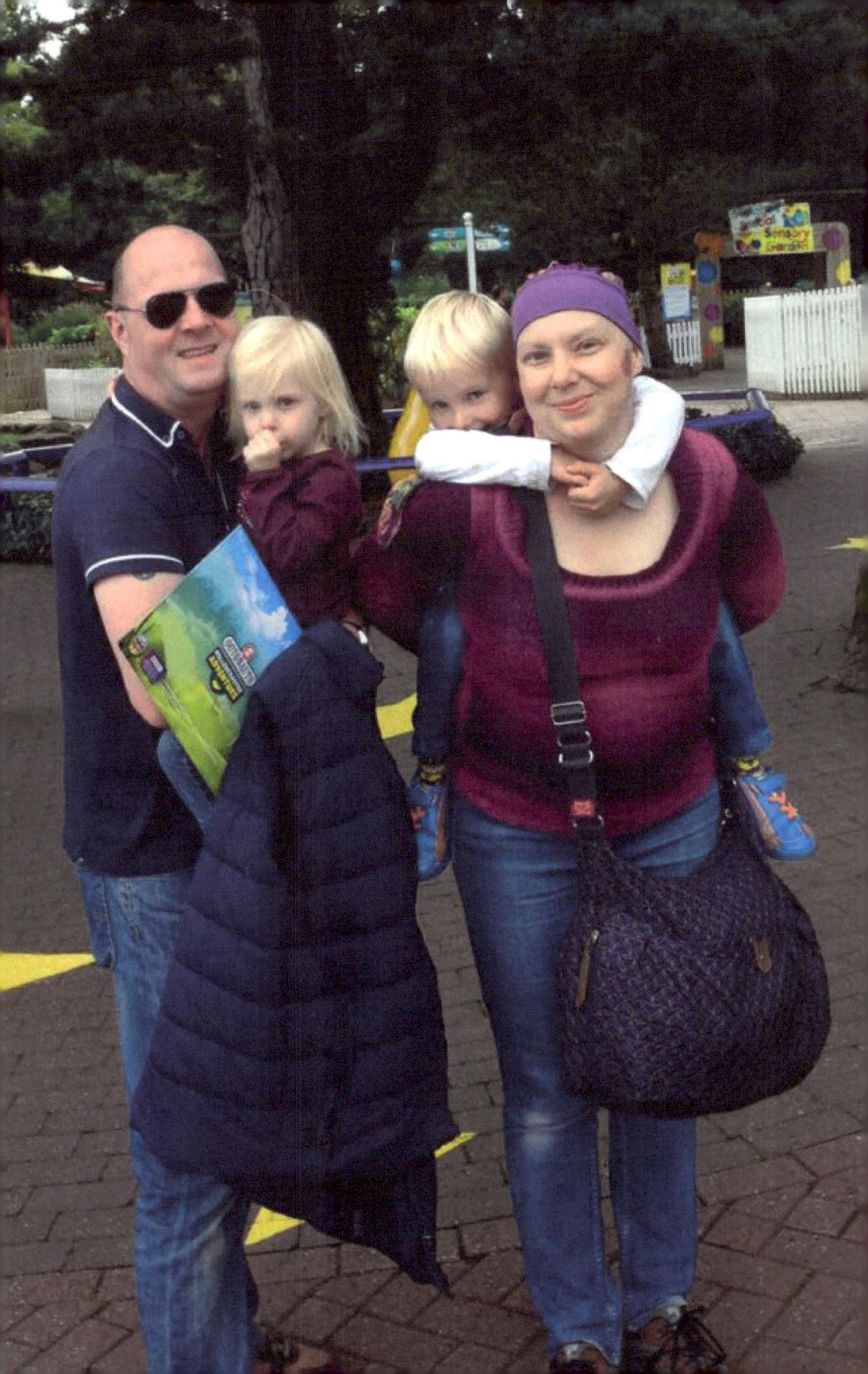

HELGA'S CHEMOTHERAPY CONTINUED, UNTIL SHE HAD COMPLETED 6 CYCLES.

THEN IT WAS TIME FOR ANOTHER SCAN, AND THE WAIT FOR THE RESULTS. THIS TIME WAS PERHAPS A LITTLE EASIER THAN THE FIRST. GIVEN CONFIDENCE BY THE FIRST POSITIVE RESULT, WE WERE LEARNING HOW TO KEEP THE FEARS AT BAY.

"LET'S NOT WORRY UNTIL WE ACTUALLY HAVE SOMETHING TO WORRY ABOUT—WE COULD WASTE ALL THIS PRECIOUS TIME WORRYING FOR NOTHING!"

THEN BEFORE YOU KNOW IT, YOU GET THE RESULT...

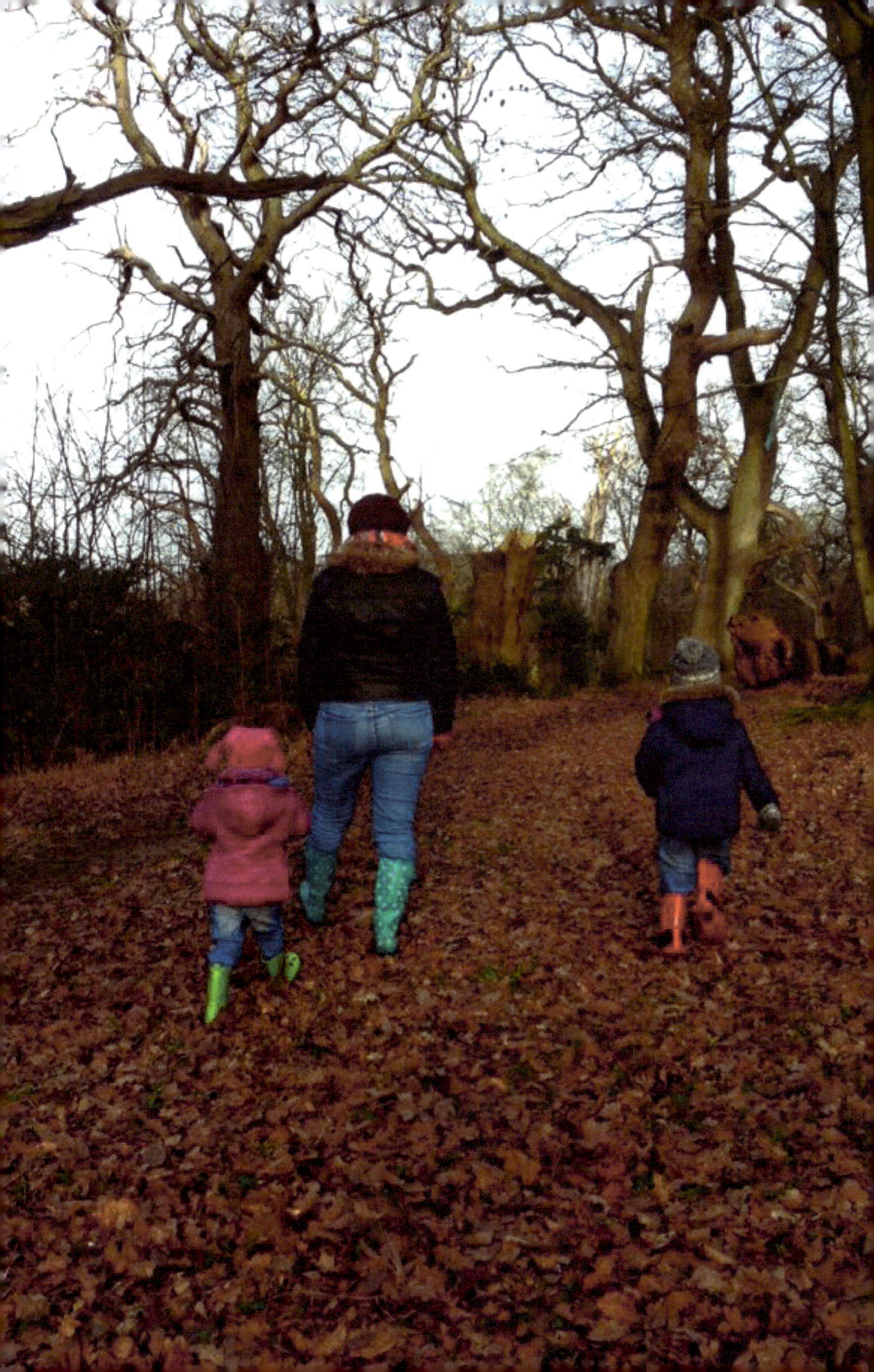

Justin Bowen updated his status
19th Oct 2016 at 18:28

A little update on Helga's treatment after seeing the specialist today. After 6 rounds of chemo the cancers have gone down dramatically. This means that she won't need to have another round of chemo, although will still get herceptin (hormone treatment) every 3 weeks. So great news!

However she will need 3 weeks of daily radiotherapy and, due to the genetic abnormality underlying her cancer, she'll still need a double mastectomy (which we expected). The surgery is scheduled for November 8th. She'll be out within a day or 2, but the recovery time will be 4-6 weeks. The radiotherapy will likely be very early January.

So all this means that although there is still a fair way to go, the bottom line is a) the treatment is going great and b) Helga should be able to enjoy a lovely Christmas.

Happy days!

❤️

ON 8TH NOVEMBER 2016, HELGA
UNDER WENT SURGERY. SHE HAD A
DOUBLE MASTECTOMY AND BREAST
RECONSTRUCTION WITH IMPLANTS. SHE
WAS FITTED WITH DRAINS TO REMOVE THE
FLUID DISCHARGE THAT WOULD FOLLOW
THE SURGERY.

Helga Peeters updated her status
9th Nov 2016 at 14:44

Thank you everyone for the many texts and messages of well wishes.

The operation went well yesterday and all to plan. I've just got a few weeks of non-driving and no lifting etc. Anyone got a spare bell?

😉

I'm now also back home with two fashionable drains in bags - that'll keep me busy a bit but I feel safer at home than at the hospital! After the recovery I found myself in a separate room on a mostly male ward. Not that this bothered me, but I did have to do a double take when a man in an operating gown was led to the toilet opposite my room by what looked like 2 prison guards, attached to one of them in a long handcuff. I kid you not!!!

😳 😂 🙈

ON 21ST NOVEMBER, HELGA HAD A
FOLLOW UP APPOINTMENT WITH HER
CONSULTANT TO SEE IF THE SURGERY HAD
BEEN SUCCESSFUL.

Helga Peeters is 😃 feeling thankful with **Justin Bowen**
21st Nov 2016 at 19:49

After months of chemo followed by surgery 2 weeks ago, I've finally had the last drain removed today. So glad to see the back of them as I kept catching them on the kitchen cupboard door handles! (Ouch!!!)

😳

Today I also had my follow up appointment with the breast surgeon checking out the new ladies. I'm up 2 brand spanking new ladies, but down 2 nipples - all looking good though.

😂👍

However also got the pathology results back on the breast tissue and lymph glands that were removed, and frankly I'm grateful we took the decision to have full clearance as the result was scary.

The left side was all clear as expected, but right breast tissue still contained 5cm of cancerous cells, even after all the chemos I'd had. On top of which out of the 16 breast lymph glands removed, 13 contained cancer rather than the 2-3 they could see on the ultrasound. It also confirmed that my cancer was fast growing.

On the upside, it's all removed now and just got recovery to get through, followed by 3 weeks of radiotherapy in January while they decide on an appropriate screening program given the rare genetic alteration and family history.

Onwards and upwards! I'm thankful for the swift NHS action which has given me a chance to hopefully watch the kids grow up and continue annoying Justin, family and all our fabulous neighbours and friends - I have no idea how we would have managed without them over these last few months!

Lots of love, *Helga*

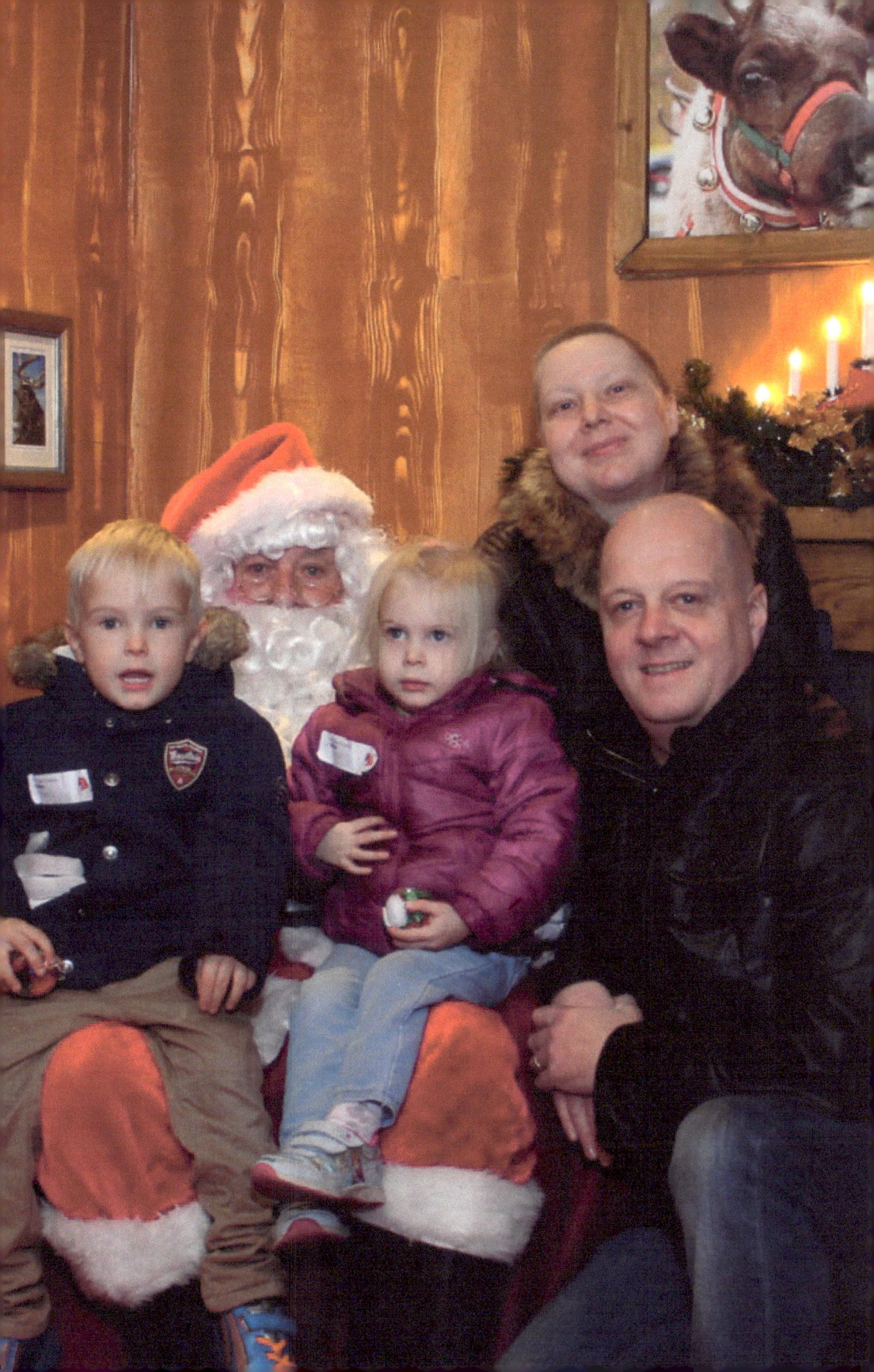

Justin Bowen updated his status
9th Dec 2016 at 20:50

This bottle of wine costs £15. It's 15% alcohol by volume and is mine. Picture number 2 is Helga's second glass. The snowman looks happy. Helga is happy. I'm sure sharing is good but this little beauty wasn't on the "Things I will share with my dear wife" list. Oh well it will soon be Christmas and she did go for her first drive today since the operation.

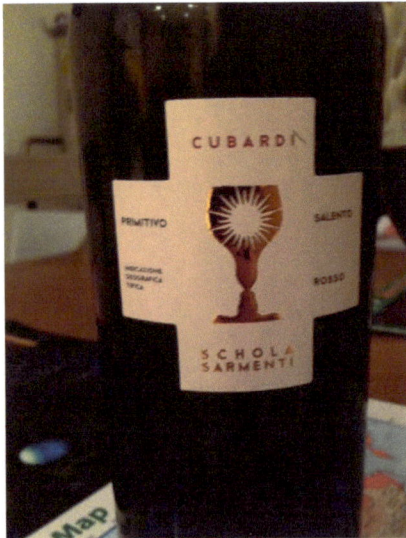

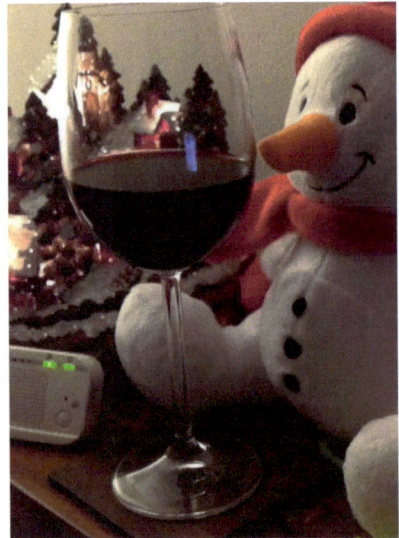

🎄 🎅 🍷

IN JANUARY 2017 HELGA HAD RADIOTHERAPY
FOR 3 WEEKS TO GET RID OF ANY REMAINING
CANCEROUS CELLS. THEN IT WAS TIME
FOR BLOOD TESTS & SCANS TO SEE IF ALL
THE TREATMENT HAD BEEN EFFECTIVE &
WHETHER SHE HAD, FOR THE TIME BEING,
"BEATEN CANCER".

Justin Bowen is 😃 feeling proud with **Helga Peeters**
15th Feb 2017 at 15:51

I've been saving this wine for a special occasion. It wasn't for Christmas or New Year or Valentine's Day. It was for today. Today is the day we got told that Helga is clear of breast cancer and THAT is the day I've been saving it for. Well done darling - I knew you'd do it!

Also just a little word to say thank you to all those who've helped us along the way. Whether it be helping out with the kids, practical stuff or just being there with love and support. You know who you are and you've all played your part. So huge thanks and appreciation and feel free to have a little celebration too in whatever way you see fit.

😀

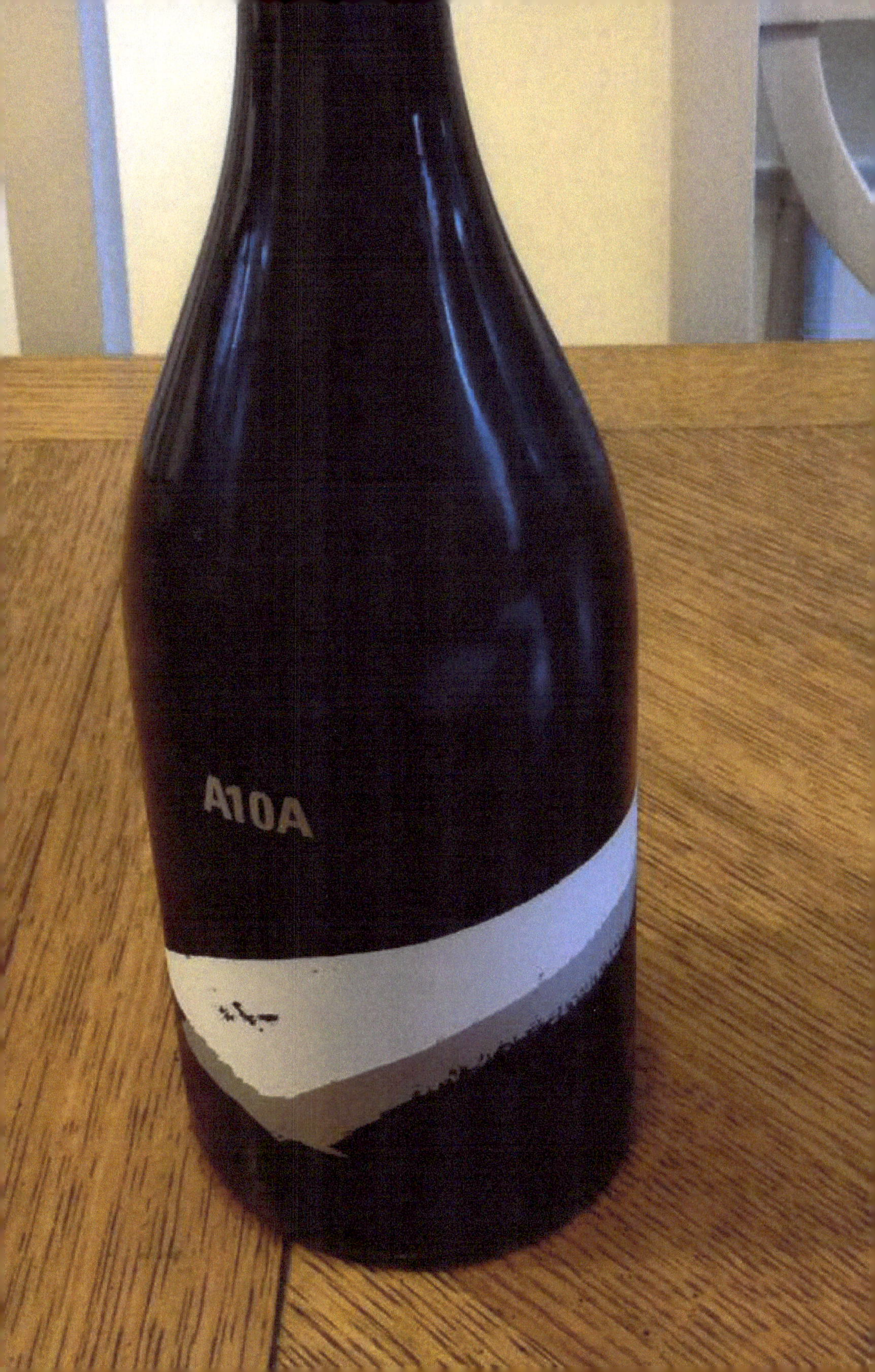
A10A

HELGA CONTINUED TO TAKE HERCEPTIN AND TAMOXIFEN TO MAKE SURE HER CANCER DIDN'T RETURN. SHE WAS BACK WORKING FULL TIME IN HER ROLE AS A FINANCIAL ANALYST. FOR SEVERAL MONTHS ALL SEEMED WELL AND LIFE RETURNED TO NORMAL. THEN IN MAY, HELGA DEVELOPED A SEVERE HEADACHE AT THE BACK OF HER HEAD. SHE INITIALLY PUT IT DOWN TO HAVING "DONE SOMETHING" TO HER NECK AT A PILATES CLASS. AS IT HADN'T GONE AFTER A COUPLE OF WEEKS, HELGA WENT TO SEE HER DOCTOR, WHO REFERRED HER FOR A SCAN.

ON 22ND MAY 2017, HELGA WENT FOR THAT SCAN. IT WAS DISCOVERED HER CANCER HAD RETURNED AND SPREAD TO HER BRAIN, RESULTING IN TWO LARGE TUMOURS. THESE WERE CAUSING HER BRAIN TO SWELL WITH FLUID.

AT THE SAME TIME, IT WAS REVEALED THAT TUMOURS HAD ALSO SPREAD TO HER LOWER ABDOMEN. THESE WERE INOPERABLE AND THEREFORE INCURABLE. HELGA WAS IMMEDIATELY ADMITTED TO UNIVERSITY HOSPITAL COVENTRY.

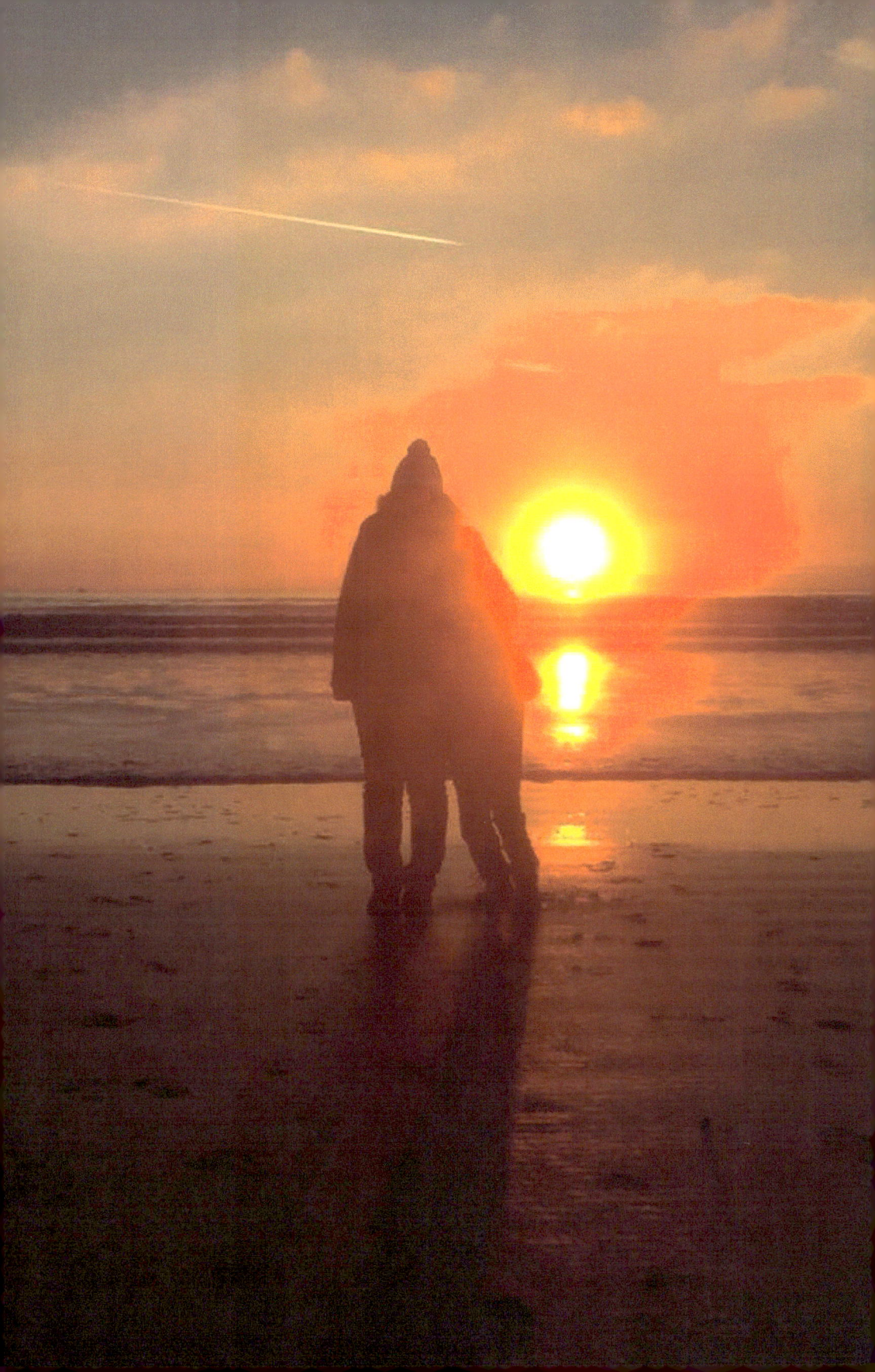

Justin Bowen is 😌 feeling ready with **Helga Peeters**
23rd May 2017 at 21:10

Life is both wonderful and brutal. It can change in an instant, whether that be by bringing unexpected joy or unleashing something so daunting that it threatens to blow you away. Families hit by the events in Manchester know this more than most today.

For us as a family, the last 24 hours have also brought us the greatest challenge. Having believed that Helga was clear of cancer, the last few months have been wonderful, with many things to be hugely positive about.

But we know now that Helga's cancer is back - and we've been told that the likelihood is that this time it can't be cured.

So, our family begins a daunting journey of unknown duration - one we will face with all the positivity and unwavering spirit we can muster.

All I ask is that you let your love and appreciation of Helga be known to her now more than ever, because now more than ever she needs it.

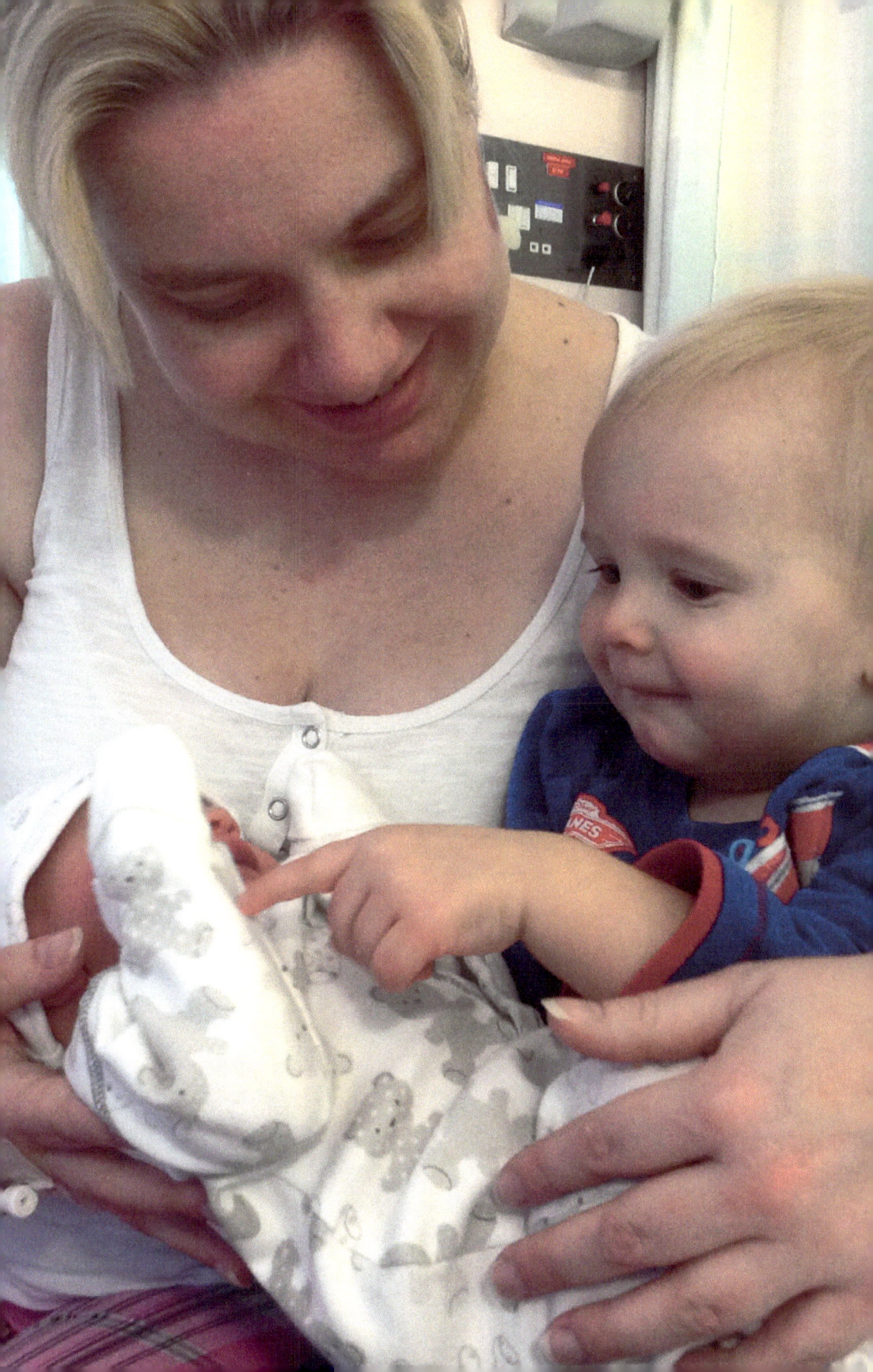

Helga Peeters
23rd May 2017 at 22:36

Not to be meant as a dark thought or anything sinister. It's merely one of my favourite quotes from The Lord of the Rings movie and I most certainly will fight till the end to delay this, but I'd like to think this quote is a beautiful thought.

#fightingforthislife

"**PIPPIN:** I DIDN'T THINK IT WOULD END THIS WAY...

GANDALF: END? NO, THE JOURNEY DOESN'T END HERE. DEATH IS JUST ANOTHER PATH, ONE THAT WE ALL MUST TAKE. THE GREY RAIN-CURTAIN OF THIS WORLD ROLLS BACK, AND ALL TURNS TO SILVER GLASS, AND THEN YOU SEE IT.

PIPPIN: WHAT? GANDALF? SEE WHAT?

GANDALF: WHITE SHORES, AND BEYOND, A FAR GREEN COUNTRY UNDER A SWIFT SUNRISE.

PIPPIN: WELL, THAT ISN'T SO BAD.

GANDALF: NO. NO IT ISN'T"

HELGA UNDERWENT EMERGENCY BRAIN SURGERY TO INSERT A TUBE (CALLED A SHUNT), WHICH WOULD DRAIN THE FLUID AND REDUCE THE SWELLING.

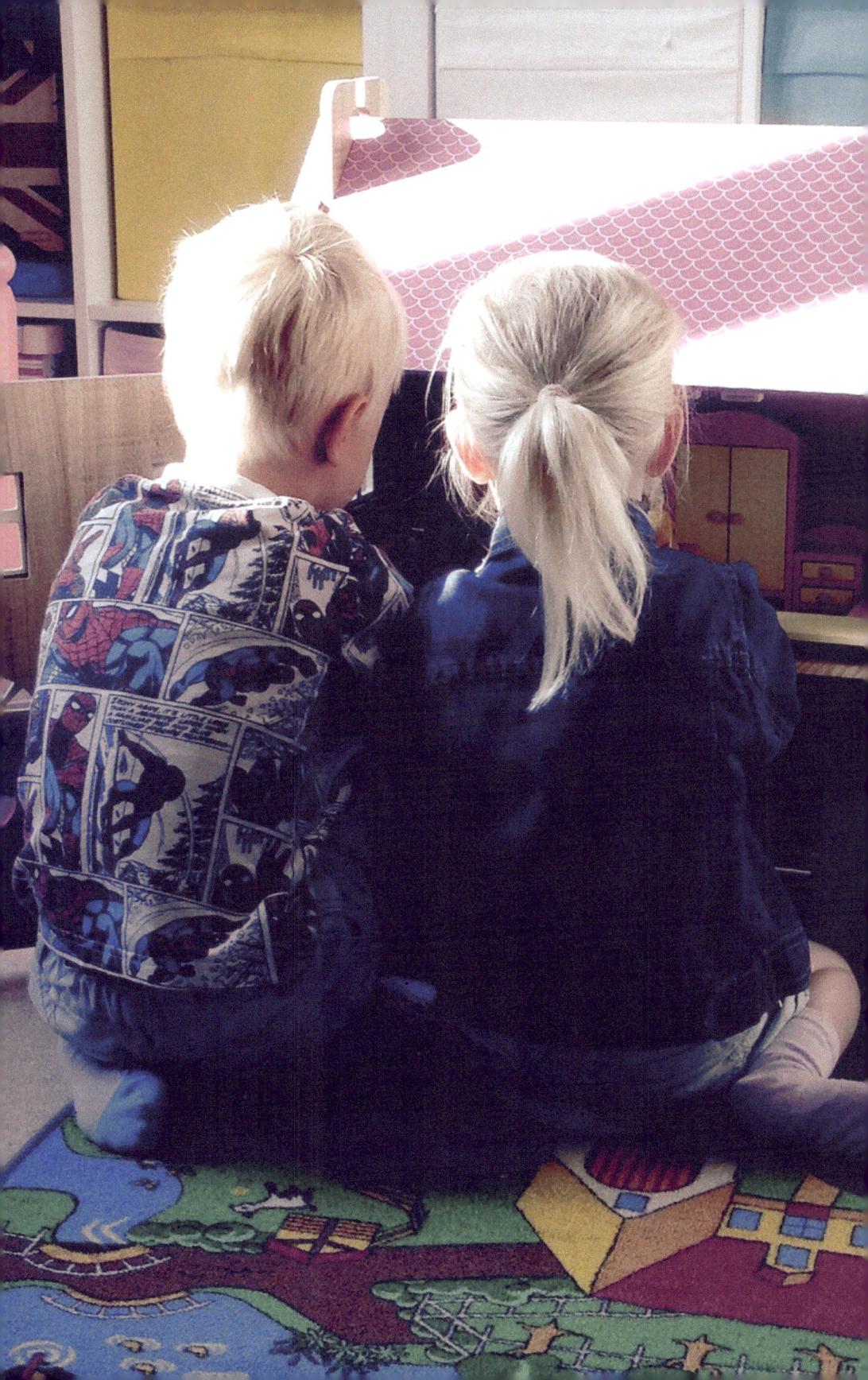

Justin Bowen is with **Helga Peeters**
26th May 2017 at 20:31

The best thing about visiting Mummy in the hospital is getting to eat all her chocolate cake!

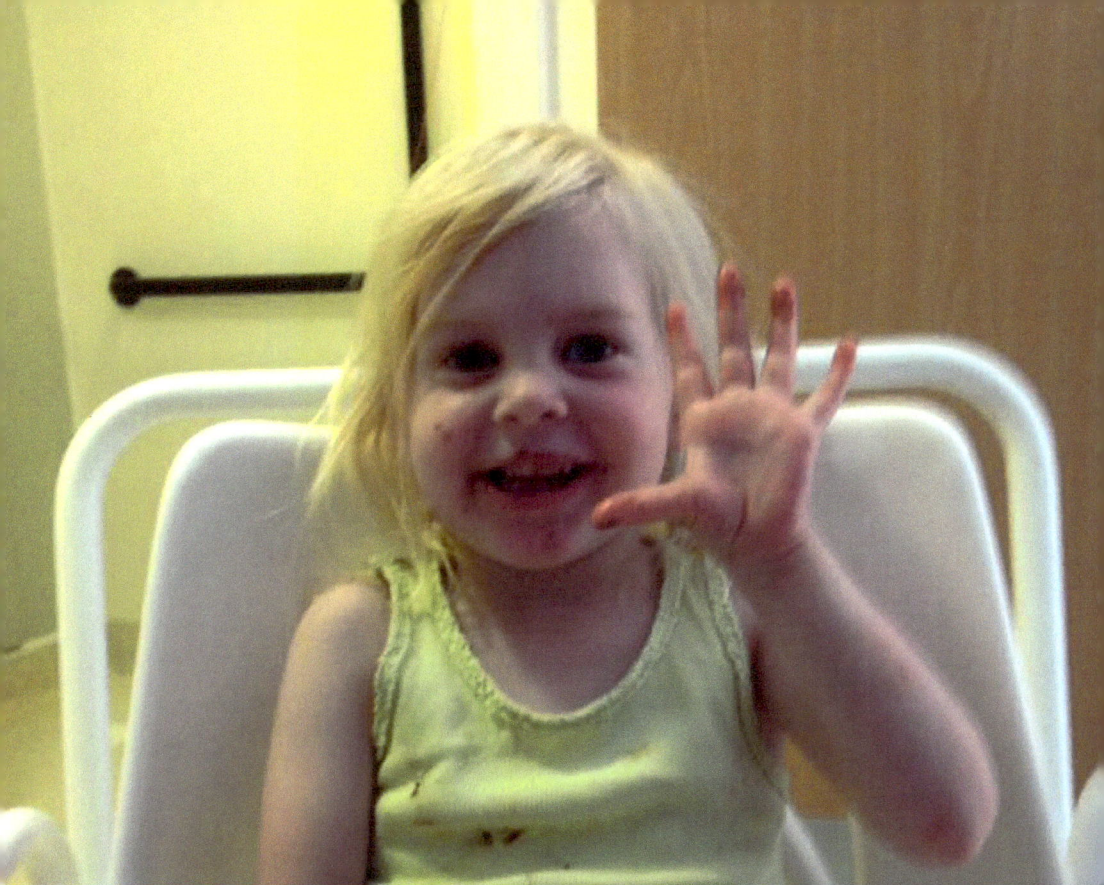

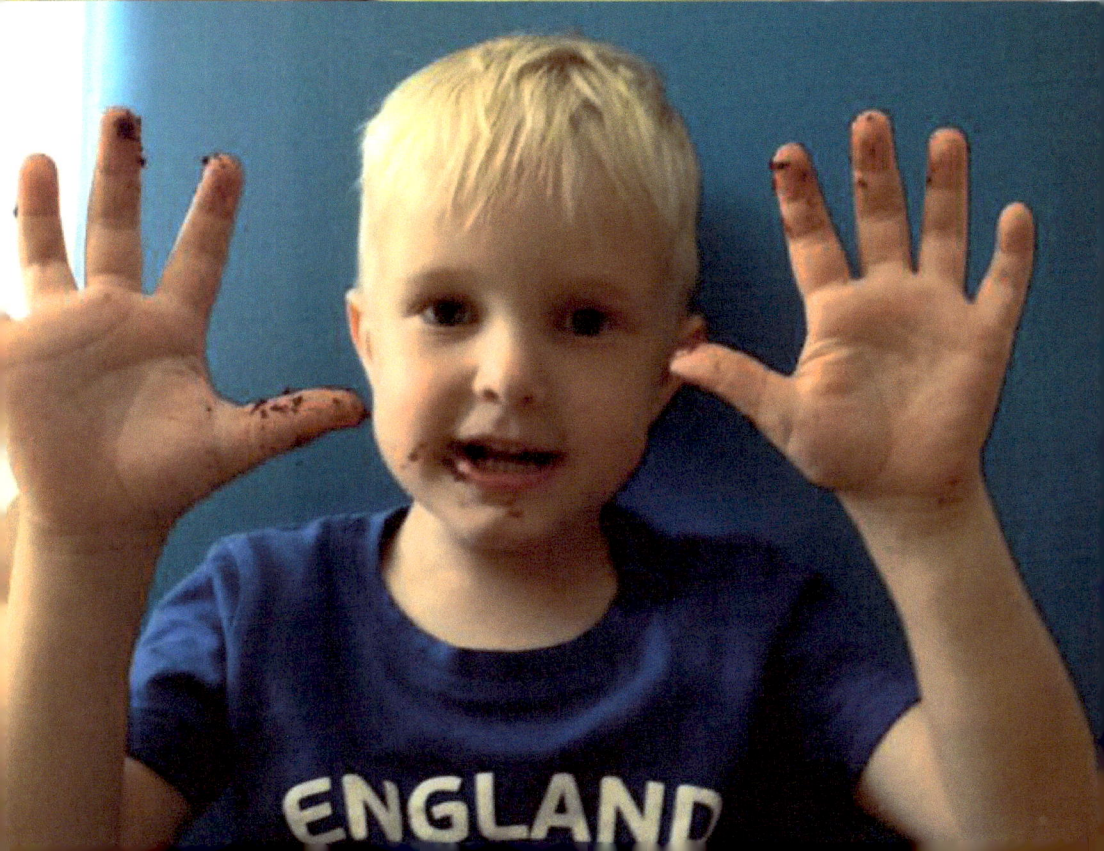

Helga Peeters
28th May 2017 at 08:30

Who knew I'd ever be found crazy enough to need to get brain surgery done?

😂

All went well, head feels much much better and tomorrow we can go home.

👍

Anyone got glow sticks and a floppy hat to match my punk hairstyle now so I can attend the rave parties?

😂🤠🤣

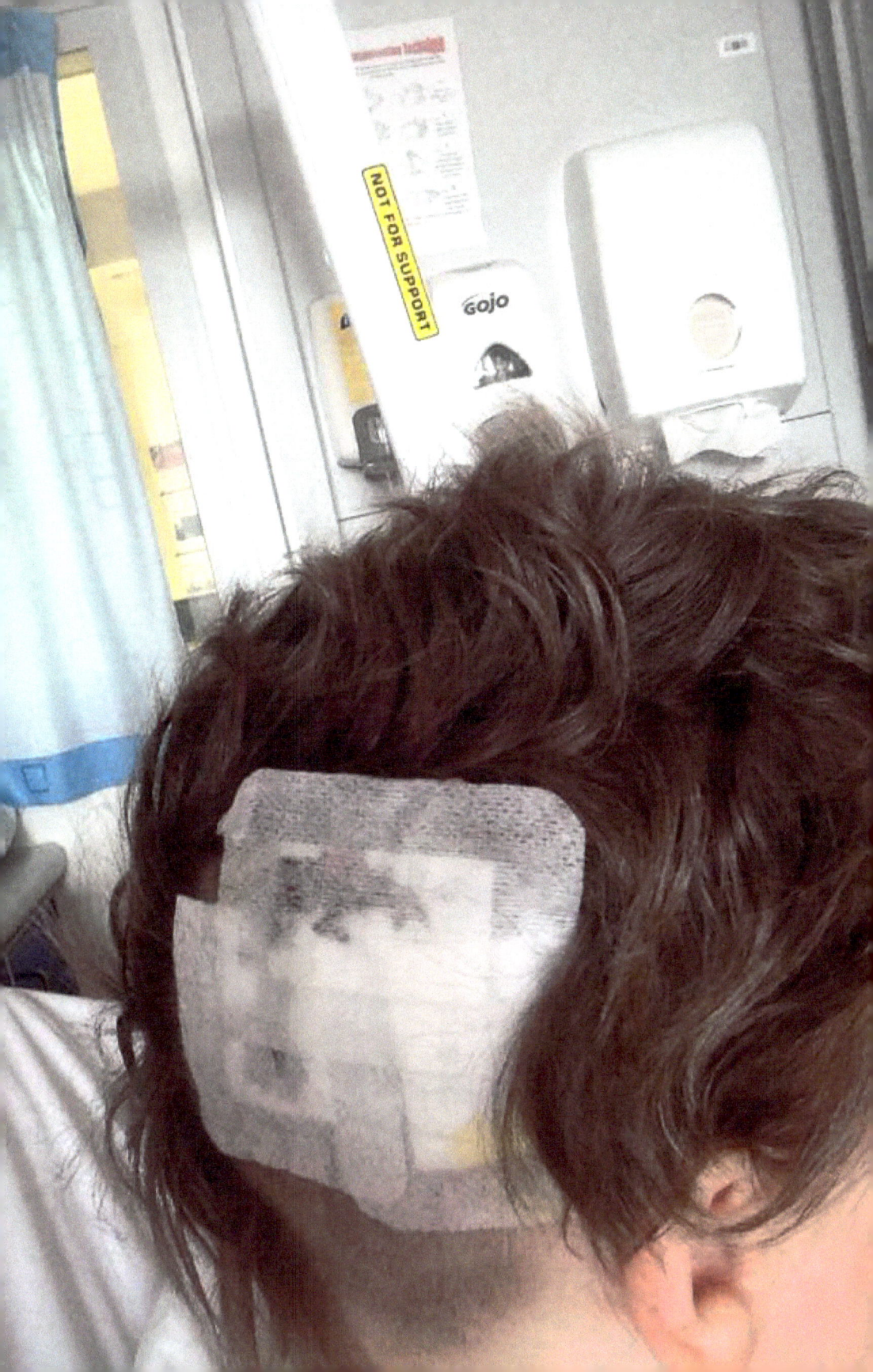

ON 30TH MAY, JUST A WEEK AFTER BEING
ADMITTED TO HOSPITAL, HELGA RETURNED
HOME. SHE HAD AN APPOINTMENT
WITH HER ONCOLOGIST AND A NEW
CHEMOTHERAPY TREATMENT WAS PLANNED
WITH A DRUG CALLED KADCYLA. THE AIM
WAS TO CONTROL THE CANCER IN HELGA'S
ABDOMEN AND AT THE SAME TIME REDUCE
THE TUMOURS IN HER BRAIN.

IF THE PLAN WORKED AND THE TUMOURS
ON HELGA'S BRAIN COULD BE SHRUNK,
HELGA WOULD THEN UNDERGO A
REVOLUTIONARY RADIOTHERAPY CALLED
CYBERKNIFE. THIS COULD POTENTIALLY
DESTROY THE BRAIN TUMOURS.

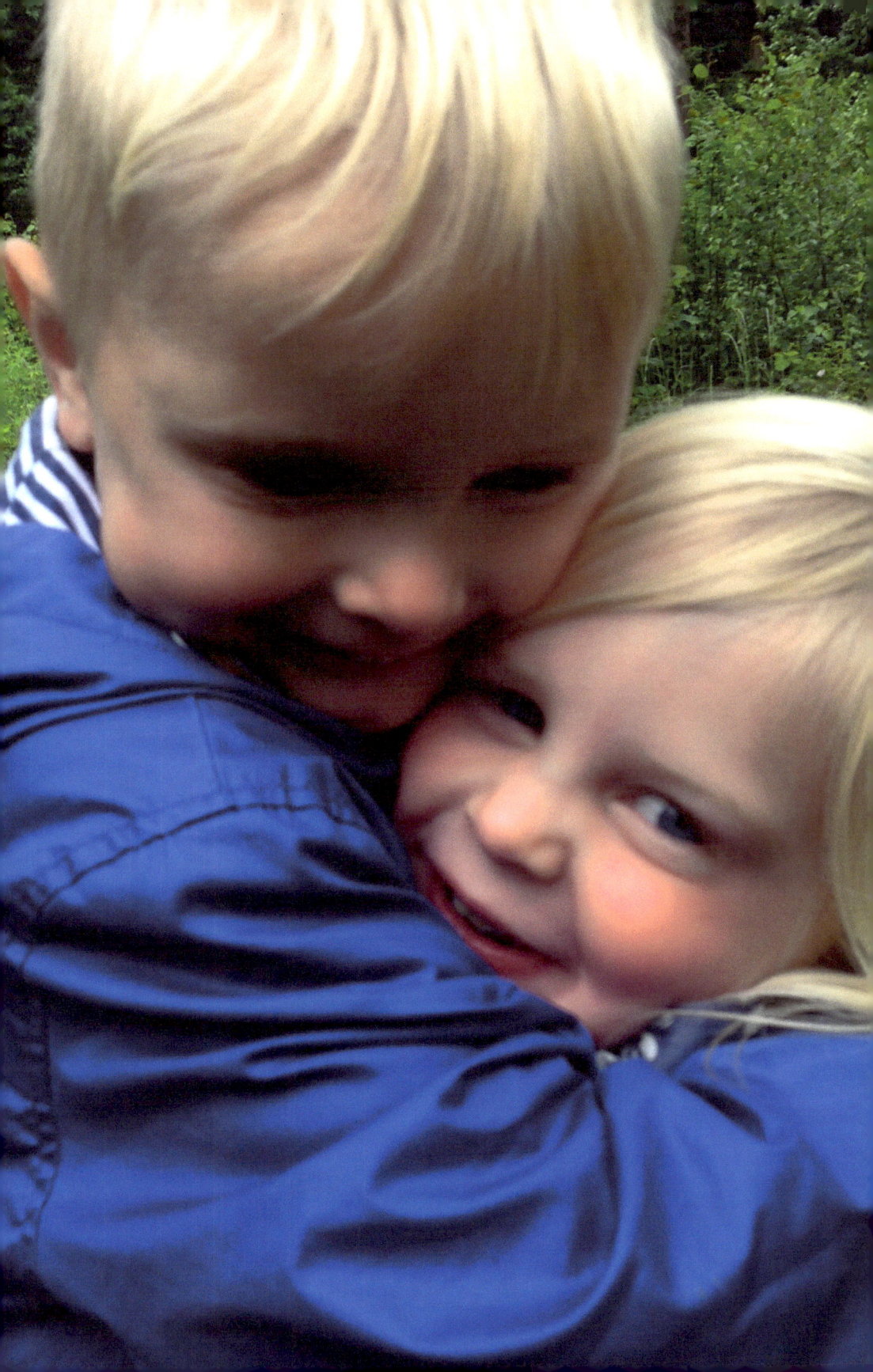

Justin Bowen is 😌 feeling accomplished with **Helga Peeters**
2nd June 2017 at 08:30

If I say so myself, that's not a bad bit of handywork with a pair of clippers!

😎

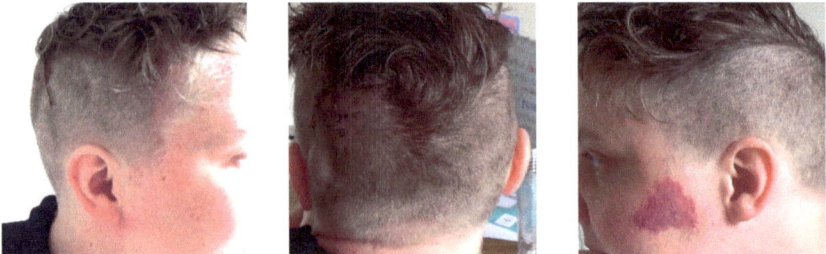

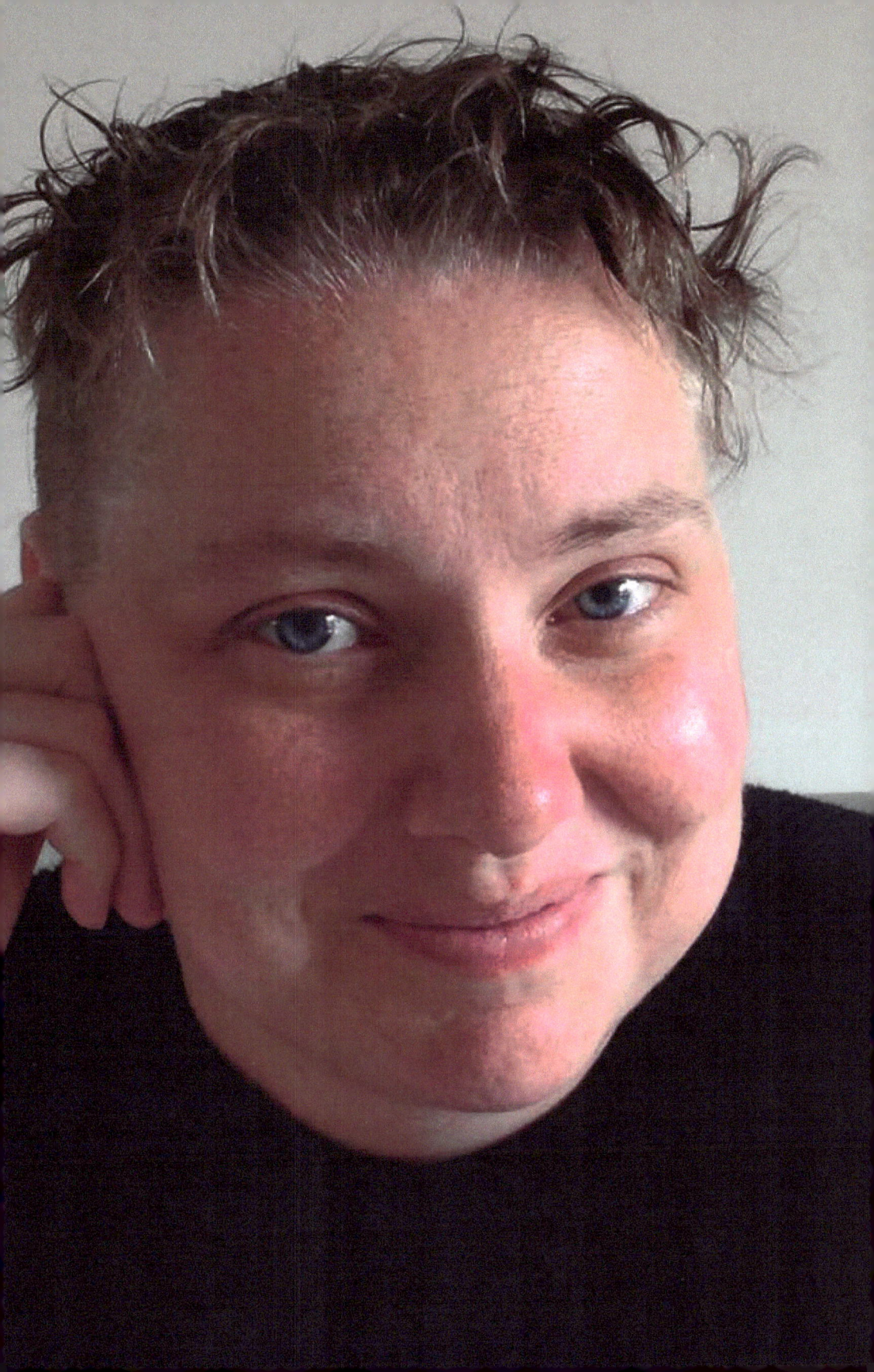

Helga Peeters
5th June 2017 at 19:10

First Kadcyla chemo happened today. Let's hope this new wonder drug does exactly for me what it's done for many others and I start feeling a bit more stable again soon.

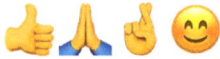

👍🙏🤞😊

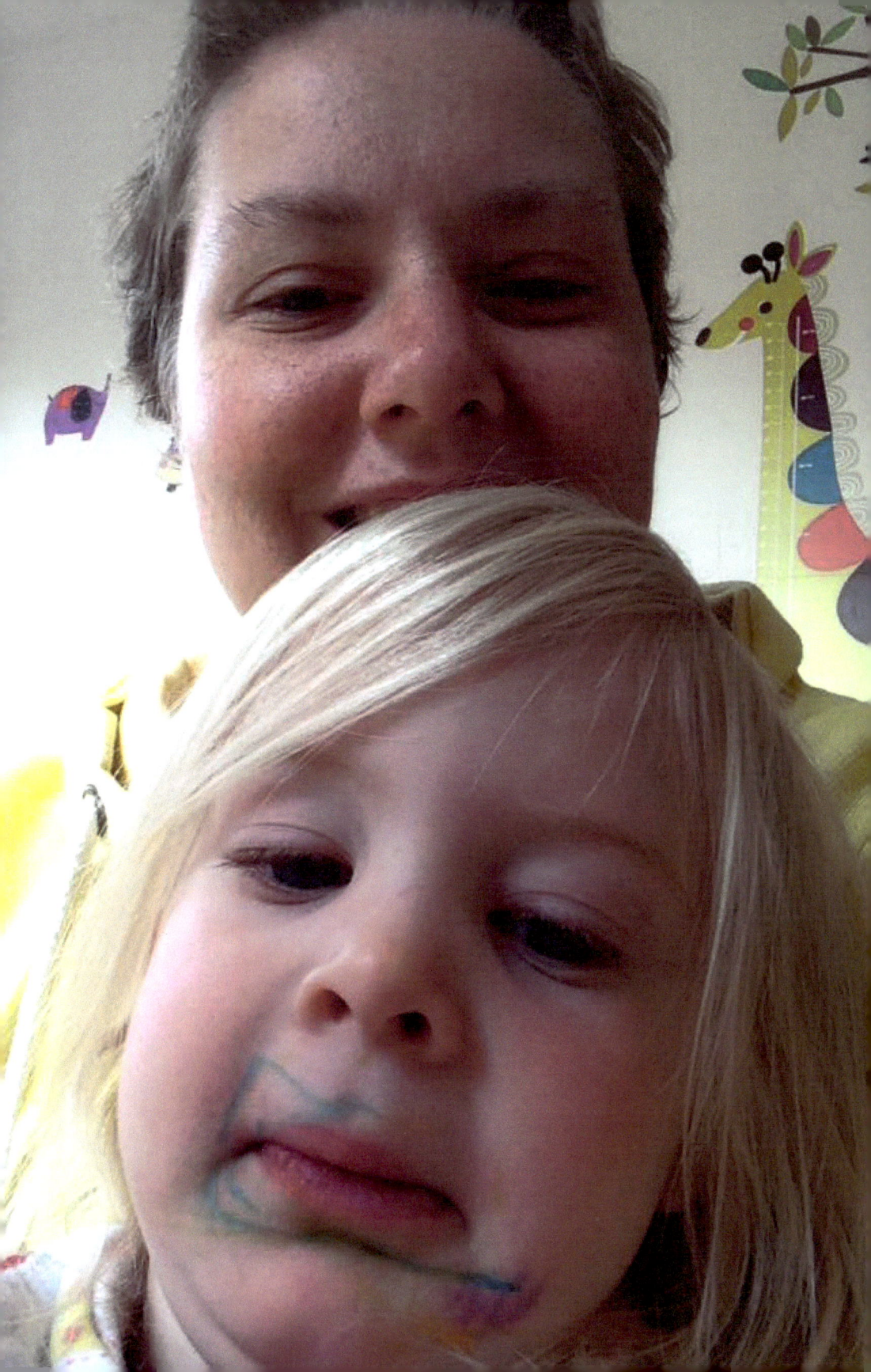

Helga Peeters
9th June 2017 at 19:10

Just to say thank you to everyone for coming to my rescue at various stages this week. I think it's fair to say my body totally hit rock bottom after they reduced some meds, and threw a new chemo on top while still recovering from the brain surgery 2 weeks ago.

After 48 hours of vomiting and being totally dehydrated we ended up in A&E being looked after by Lorna's amazing team. And they pieced me back together bit by bit over 24 hours.

We're stronger again and for the first time in weeks I actually feel 70- 80% again myself. So hopefully we're on the way up again now.

Thank you for the rescue drivers Tom and Anna.
Where would I be without you lot?

😘

And as always a special thanks to Justin for just being amazing and picking up all the pieces while I was 'awol'.

Thank you all for the messages etc, apologies I've not responded to them all xx

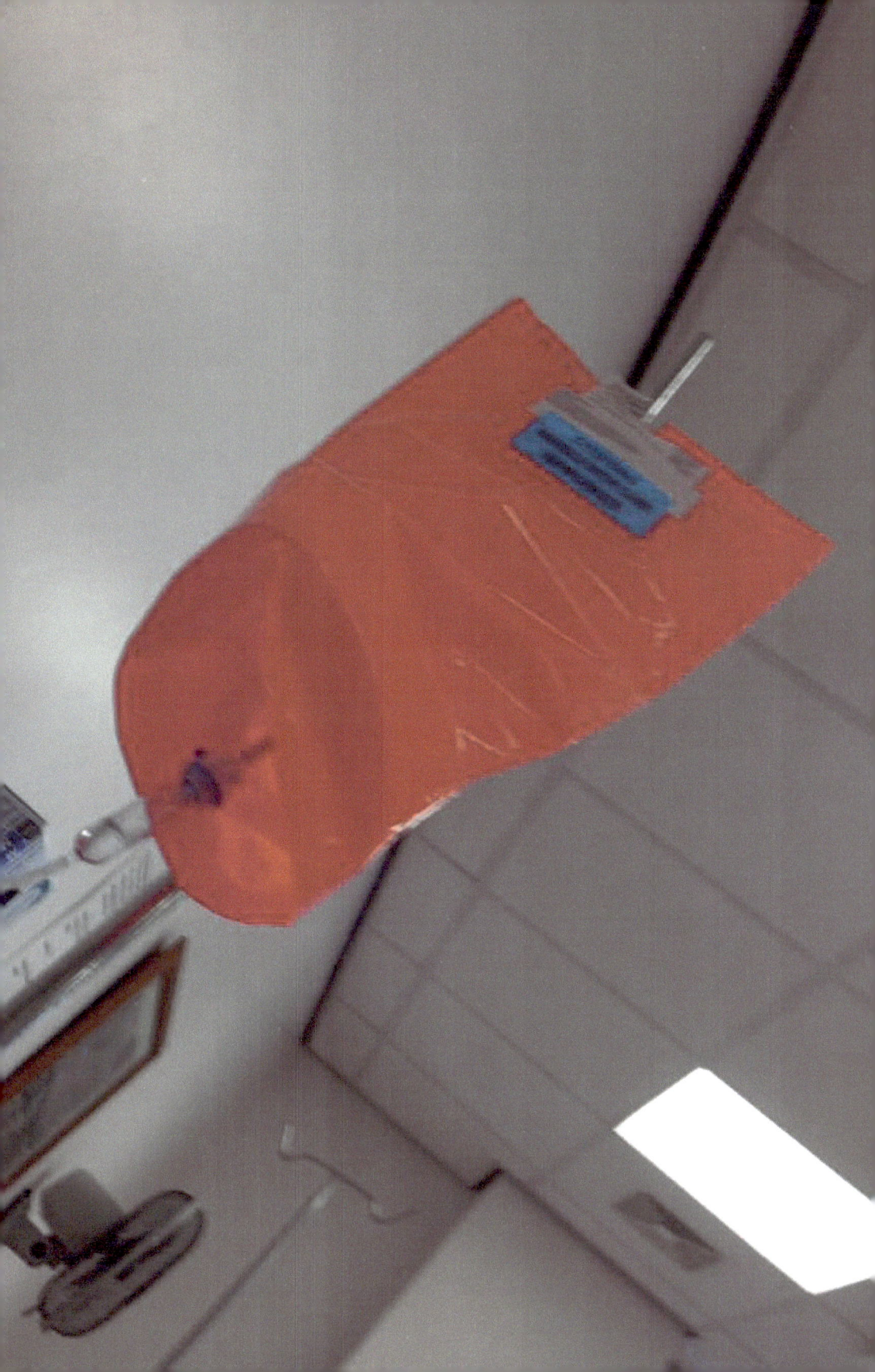

AFTER SOME INITIAL PROBLEMS, MAINLY DUE TO THE AFTER EFFECTS OF BRAIN SURGERY, HELGA'S NEW TREATMENT WENT WELL AND THE FIRST SCAN SHOWED A SIGNIFICANT REDUCTION IN THE SIZE OF THE BRAIN TUMOURS. ON 15TH JULY 2017 WE CELEBRATED OUR 10TH WEDDING ANNIVERSARY.

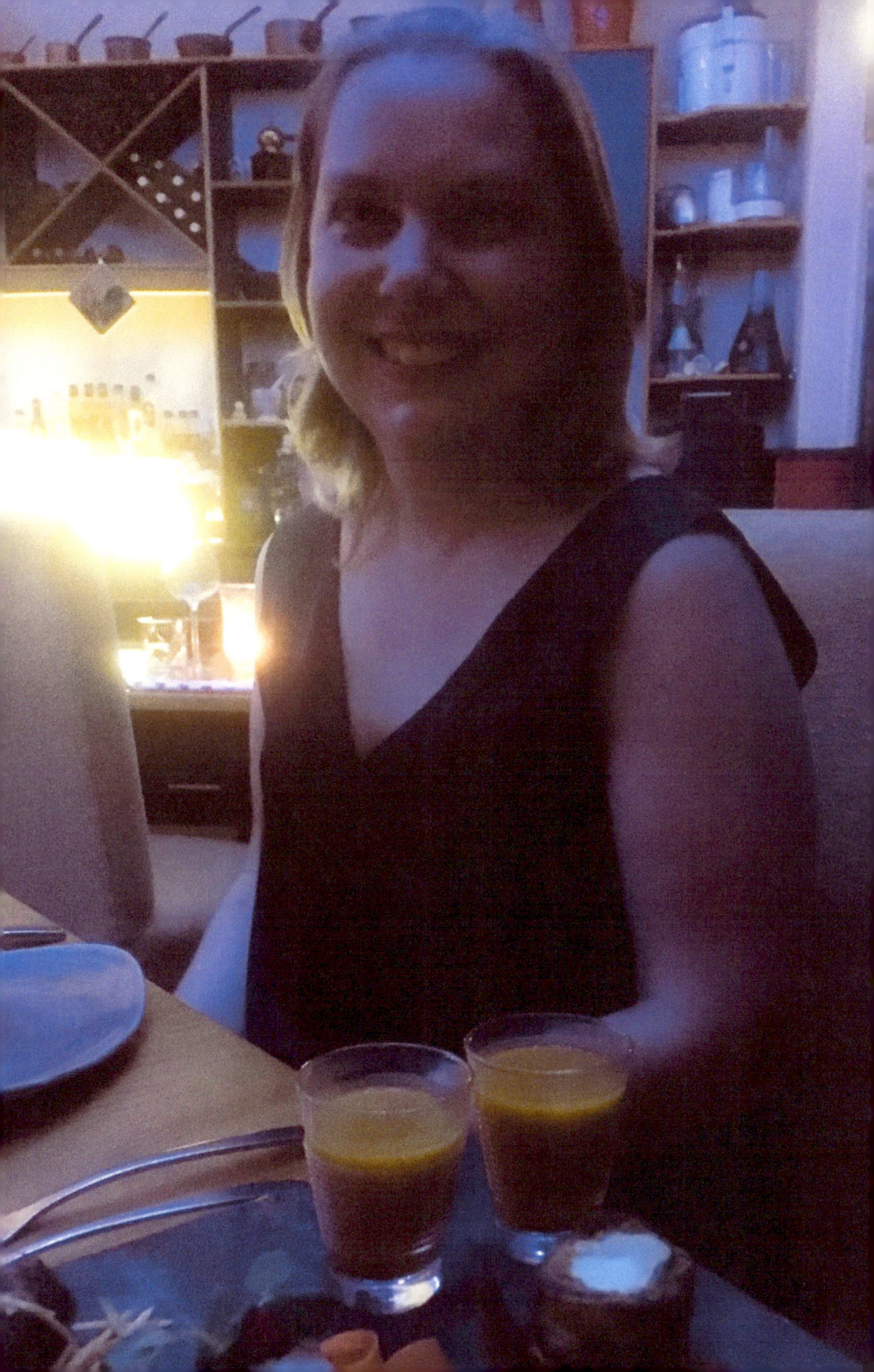

Helga Peeters is with **Justin Bowen**
15th July 2017 at 08:06

Happy 10th Anniversary to the best husband and friend I could wish for. We've had our major challenges within that timeframe but got through it, so here's hoping I can do another 10-20 more at least!

Love you lots!!

❤️

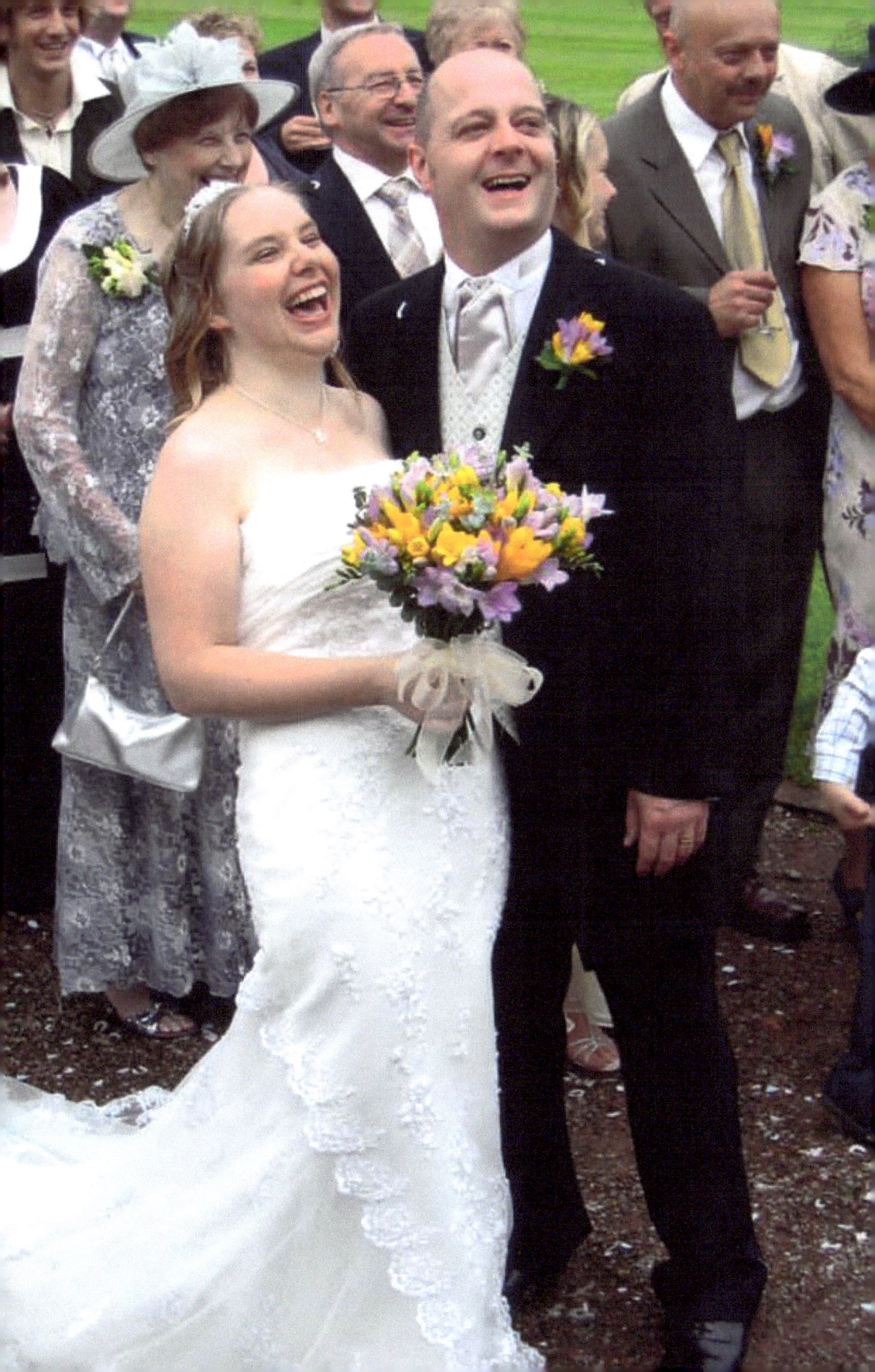

THE TREATMENT CONTINUED AND
KADCYLA PROVED TO BE HUGELY EFFECTIVE
IN SHRINKING THE TUMOURS ON HELGA'S
BRAIN. IT WAS ALSO CONTROLLING THE
TUMOURS IN HER ABDOMEN. IN SEPTEMBER,
HELGA UNDERWENT CYBERKNIFE
TREATMENT ON HER BRAIN TUMOURS AT
QUEEN ELIZABETH HOSPITAL, BIRMINGHAM.
THIS WAS FOLLOWED BY SCANS AND, TWO
WEEKS LATER, AN APPOINTMENT TO FIND
OUT WHETHER ALL THE TREATMENT HAD
BEEN EFFECTIVE.

Helga Peeters is 🙂 feeling relieved with **Justin Bowen**
6th Oct 2017 at 16:10

As I stand before the evening of my 35th, I reflect and celebrate all the good that has come from the bad cards I've been dealt.

I feel blessed to be surrounded by so many good friends, family and neighbours who at times have picked the pieces of me up and put them back together. It means more to me than I could ever put into words! You keep me sane and make it all worthwhile.

Over the last 4 months, I've been told I'm 'stage 4 incurable' (treatable, yes, but never to be cured), put on Kadcyla, had brain surgery, had cyberknife and seen the inside of more machines spread over different hospitals than I can count on 1 hand (I think they like to keep me fit or keep public transport in business!), but now it's been found the treatment is working an absolute treat and keeping control of the cancer - for now.

The lymph glands in my abdomen have gone back to their normal size and the brain tumors are now less than half the size of what they were, leaving just dead tissue in my brain. (Always knew there were question marks about dead brain cells!)

🙂

So what's next I hear you all ask? We keep going with this beauty Kadcyla until there's a day it either stops working or I'm considered stable enough to take the leap of faith to come off it and see how long it lasts before it rears its ugly head again. (May both these options be far away into the future still while my mental state finds peace again in the fragile cancer world.)

Meanwhile, I'll be having cake and prosecco tonight to celebrate and leave you all in peace with the message: 'As it's breast cancer October, check yourselves and get anything suspicious checked out. Facebook games/status hearts etc really do nothing. But don't take my word for it!'

HELGA CONTINUED THE CYCLE OF TAKING
KADCYLA AND HAVING HER CANCER
MONITORED THROUGH THE REST OF 2017
AND INTO THE NEW YEAR.

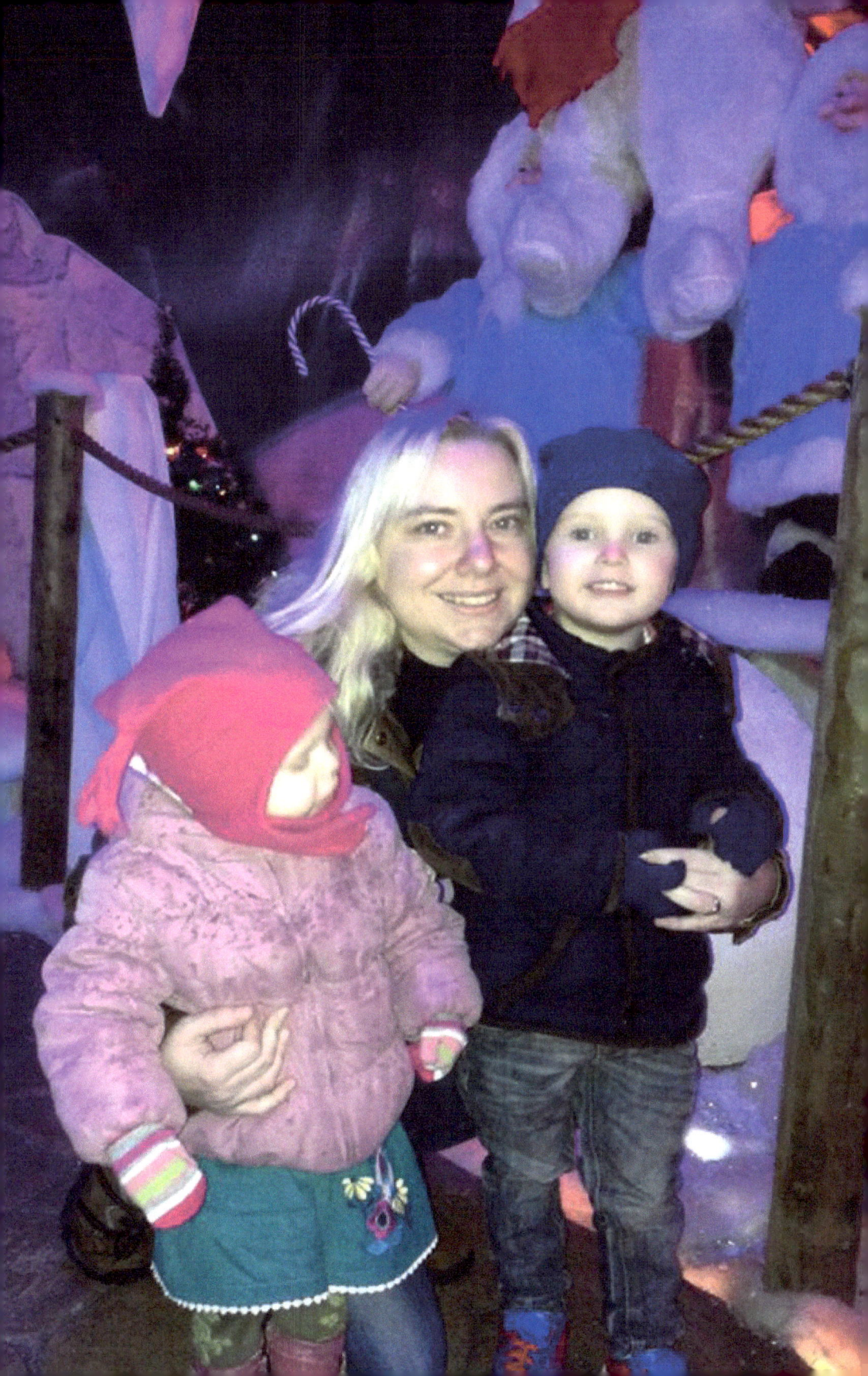

Justin Bowen is with **Helga Peeters** at **Monkwood Green**
31st Dec 2017 at 15:56

One last walk to see out 2017. What a year that's been!
So here's to an uneventful, slighty dull but exceedingly happy 2018!

❤️

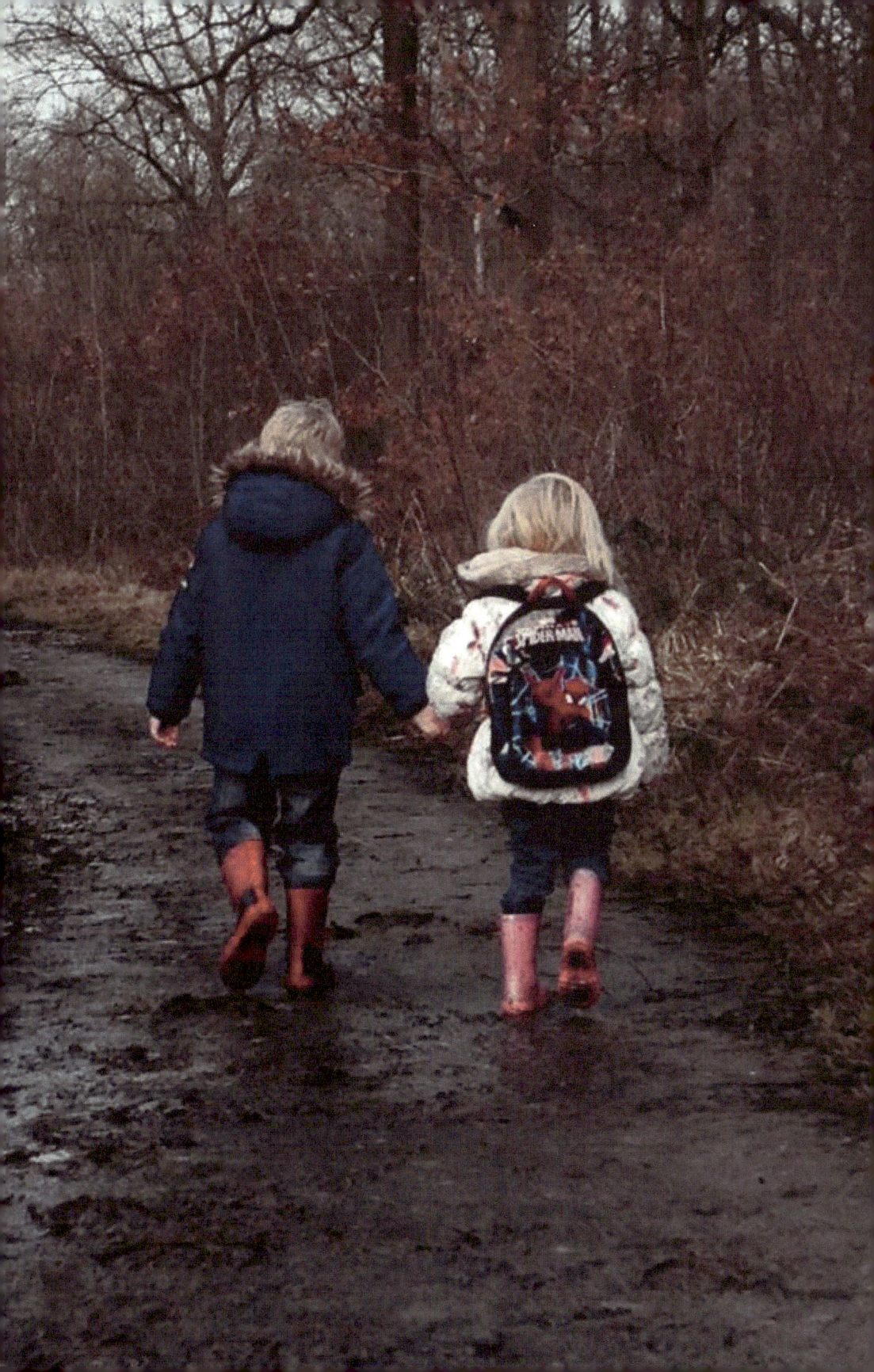

Helga Peeters is 😇 feeling blessed with **Justin Bowen**
31st Jan 2018 at 19:54

My apologies for not having done an update for a long time, but we got into a bit of a routine with 3-weekly treatments, starting work again etc.

Since May, life with stage 4 cancer (incurable/advanced/metastatic stage) has been a rollercoaster. I'm on 3-weekly Kadcyla 'for life', or at least until the day it stops working and keeping the cancer spread at bay. Luckily apart from 2 days of tiredness, it is side effect free. No hair loss, no sickness etc.

We knew from the full body scan in December that it was working nicely and had reversed the damage done to my abdomen lymph glands, as well as having reduced the brain tumours a lot. Yesterday we had the first check up since the cyberknife treatment at the end of September and I'm pleased to inform you all there isn't a spot to be seen anywhere whatsoever - just a bit of black shading from dead cell remnants where the biggest tumour was. (Doubt I've actually used those ones anyway!)

😂

The long and short of it is we live to fight another day, being in complete remission. I could have hugged the consultant earlier!

So, while we're having a calm before the next storm (may that storm be many years away while chemo is working a treat), I gazed upon the sky on the train earlier, smiling and filled with joy. I am having a celebratory cocktail (yep it looks green but it's blue caracao, vodka and orange juice!) and counting my blessings in this life as I know at the other end of the scale are those whose treatments have stopped working.

Cheers all!

🥂

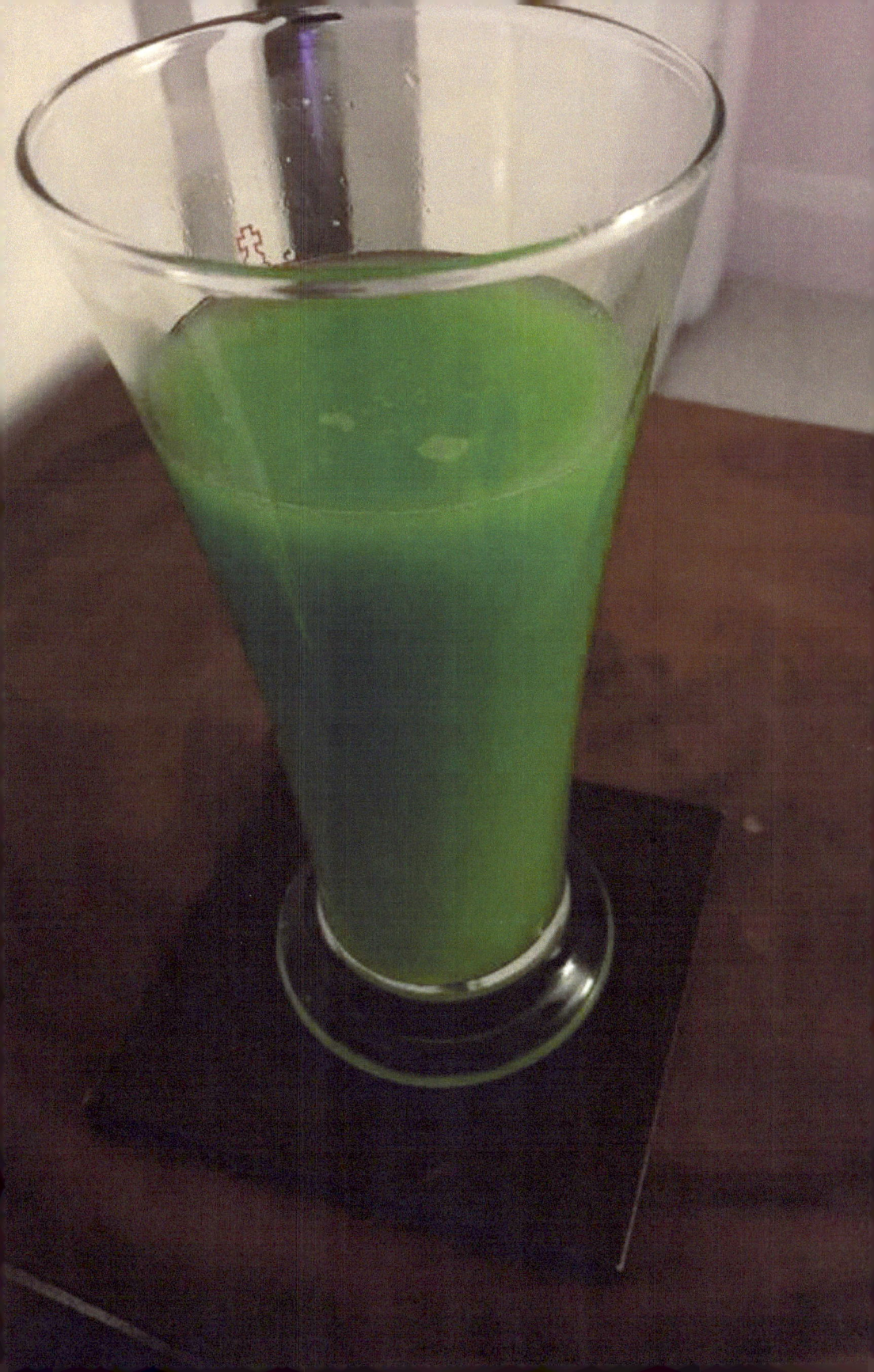

TREATMENT CONTINUED THROUGH
FEBRUARY 2018 AND AT THE BEGINNING
OF MARCH HELGA WENT FOR THE NEXT
SCAN. AGAIN THE WAIT. ALTHOUGH
OUR CONFIDENCE HAD BEEN SHAKEN
BY THE EVENTS OF THE PREVIOUS YEAR,
WE REMAINED POSITIVE AND OUR WELL
PRACTICED ROUTINES TO MANAGE THE
"SCANXIETY" WERE PUT INTO PLAY. THE
THING IS ANY OUTCOME IS POSSIBLE, SO
YOU LITERALLY HAVE NO IDEA WHAT IS
GOING TO HAPPEN. EQUALLY, BY THIS STAGE
OUR RESOLVE NOT TO WASTE PRECIOUS
MOMENTS WORRYING ABOUT SOMETHING
WE COULDN'T CONTROL WAS ABSOLUTE.
BESIDES, YOU FIND OUT SOON ENOUGH...

Helga Peeters is 🙁 feeling nervous with **Justin Bowen**
19th March 2018 at 17:19

The jury is in on the results.

The good news, it has not mutated. It's still HER2 positive which means in common terms that a lot of the targeted options remain available to control/treat it.

The bad news, Kadcyla has stopped working for me after 7-8 months which is a shame because it was such an easy and tolerable chemo for me and did wonders on my brain tumours.

So, new treatment plan is back on herceptin on its own (like before my Kadcyla), but I'll have a combination of 2 chemos called GemCarbo which apparently have given proven results on girls with the BRCA mutations. So hopefully as my PALB2 mutation is closely linked to them, it will work well for me too.

As for side effects that's to be 'wait and see' as it can hit hard on the immune system due to low white bloods and low platelets. Yet others have sailed through it.

🤷‍♀️

I'm expecting I'm going to react somewhere in the middle to 2 years ago where the chemos wiped me out and my easy Kadcyla.

Fingers crossed and just shows the success of us pushing for extra screening rather than waiting for symptoms to appear before anything gets investigated.

🤔 😳

AND SO ANOTHER ROUND OF TREATMENT
BEGAN, THIS TIME WITH GEMCARBO. THIS
TREATMENT WAS HARDER ON HELGA THAN
THE KADCYLA HAD BEEN. FROM HAVING
VIRTUALLY NO SIDE-EFFECTS PREVIOUSLY,
THE NEW DRUG TOOK ITS TOLL ON HER
IMMUNE SYSTEM. THIS MEANT LOTS OF
ADDITIONAL VISITS TO THE HOSPITAL AND
TINKERING WITH THE DOSAGE, TRYING
TO FIND A LEVEL THAT HER BODY COULD
STAND. IT'S ONE OF THE CHALLENGES OF
CHEMOTHERAPY - THE DRUG MAY WELL
BE EFFECTIVE ON THE CANCER, BUT YOUR
BODY HAS TO BE ABLE TO SUSTAIN THE
TREATMENT. GRADUALLY A MANAGEABLE
BALANCE WAS FOUND AND BEFORE LONG IT
WAS "THAT" TIME AGAIN.

Helga Peeters is 😕 feeling relaxed with **Justin Bowen**
9th June 2018 at 09:39

The results are in from the full ct scan, well mostly...

Lymph glands of my abdomen have vastly improved so the GemCarbo is working really well on it.

As for the head, they are getting a 2nd opinion from QE Birmingham by the cyberknife team because Worcester didn't have the January scan to compare with (which showed the scarring and dead cells from cyberknife). So as they are comparing to a September scan prior to cyberknife they are putting the shades down as cancerous when likelihood is that it's dead cells.

If it was cancerous my headaches would be on the same scale again as last year prior to the shunt put in, so he/me aren't worried as such...for now. Sooo, a small sigh of relief hoping the treatments settle down again and we can fall into another routine.

One thing I will need to get done is get a Hickman-line inserted as my veins are giving up in my left arm from everything.

Whatever makes life easier hey...

😉

THE 2ND OPINION ON HELGA'S BRAIN SCAN
WAS POSITIVE. THE SHADING ON HER BRAIN
WAS DEAD RATHER THAN CANCEROUS CELLS,
SO THE TREATMENT WITH GEMCARBO
CONTINUED. IT WAS TAKING ITS TOLL ON
HELGA'S BODY, BUT SHE COMPLETED 6
CYCLES. AFTER THAT IT WAS DECIDED TO
STOP TREATMENT TO LET HER IMMUNE
SYSTEM RECOVER.

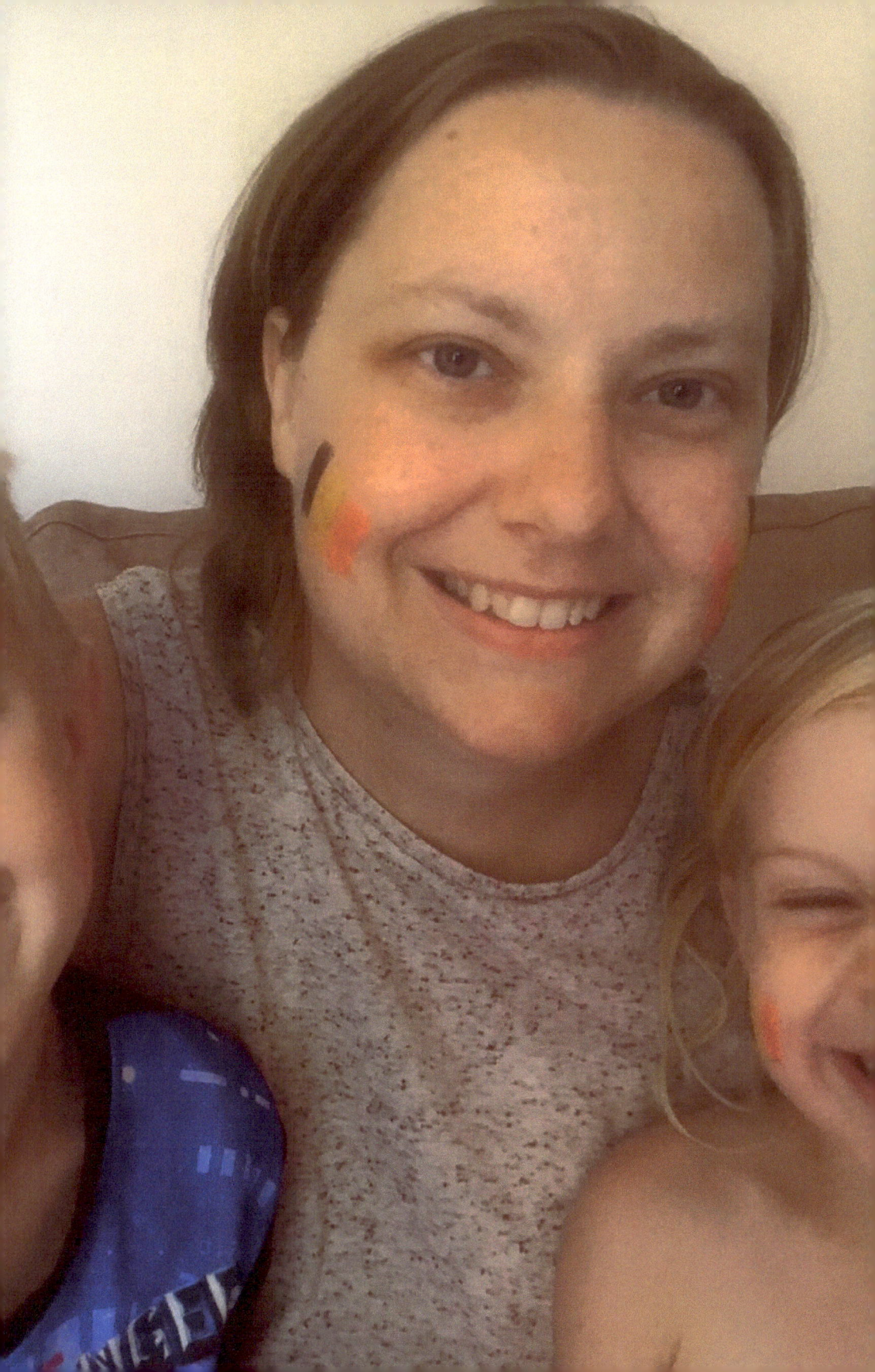

Helga Peeters is 😊 feeling relaxed with **Justin Bowen**
9th June 2018 at 09:39

Last chemo today. I can't say I won't be sorry to see the back of them for a while!! What's next I hear you say? A bloody long holiday!

😂

No in all seriousness, at least a three month break. My body (bonemarrow in particular) simply can't take any more. If they push more cycles of this GemCarbo on me then my body will completely give up and on a long-term basis I wouldn't be able to have any further treatment.

So, 3 month break from treatments and then a scan to see how my body is doing. All being well it shows a stable scan/negligible progression at best and I'll get another 3 months off. Should the scan come back with lots of progression without treatments, I'll go onto plan B (C-Z? Kind of lost track of where I got up to).

🤔

Feel a bit like my safety net is being taken away as I've had non-stop chemo/monitoring for 13 months. However at least that's being replaced with 3-monthly scans to keep an eye on whether intervention is required.

Different schedule, different way of living again... by the words of Dori (Finding Nemo) "just keep swimming"

AS HELGA'S VEINS HAD BECOME DAMAGED
OVER THE TWO YEARS SHE'D BEEN
RECEIVING TREATMENT, IN JULY 2018 SHE
HAD A HICKMAN LINE INSERTED. THIS IS
A CATHETER WHICH ALLOWS BLOOD TO
BE TAKEN AND ALSO CHEMOTHERAPY TO
BE GIVEN. IT NEEDS TO BE CLEANED OUT
EVERY WEEK TO PREVENT INFECTION SO,
EVERY THURSDAY, WE'D GO TO OUR LOCAL
COMMUNITY HOSPITAL WHERE HELGA'S
HICKMAN WOULD BE "FLUSHED OUT". IT
WAS THE ONLY TIME WHEN I HEARD HELGA
COMPLAIN ABOUT HER TREATMENT. I
WASN'T SURE WHETHER IT WAS HAVING
TO GO EVERY WEEK AND SHE SAW IT AS AN
INCONVENIENCE IN HER BUSY SCHEDULE
(SHE WAS STILL WORKING) OR WHETHER
SHE MISSED THE CAMARADERIE OF THE
ONCOLOGY WARD - I SUSPECT IT WAS A
COMBINATION OF EVERYTHING.

Helga Peeters
24th August 2018 at 11:37

The best and worst of the NHS. As good as the staff have always been for the past 2 years, so it was questionable today.

Line flushing needed by the district nurses (that's a whole palava in itself rather than the excellent care I've been getting at Worcester) and I know she didn't mean bad in any way...

Sat finally outside the right room waiting for a good half hour with nobody to be seen (this is after getting sent round the hospital in Bromsgrove because nobody seemed to know where to go), finally a nurse turns up and the following happened:

Nurse: Oh you're not what I expected! I was expecting someone alot older!
Me: Looking rather puzzled so nurse looks at the name on my notes I was carrying.
Nurse: Oh yeah, Helga, you are next - yeah so I have got the right one. You're totally not what I was expecting. What are you here for?
Me: (still looking rather puzzled) Err a line flush?
Nurse: So what have you got it in for?
Me: Stage 4 cancer treatment
Nurse: How long have you had that then?
Me: 2 years
Nurse: What did you have done then?
Me: Summing up the past 2 years as she wanted to know every detail...
Nurse: So you got a genetic mutation (guessed that without mentioning)
Me: I've got the rare one PALB2 yes
Nurse: Oh, so not even the standard BRCA ones? So you always knew you were bound to get it?
Me: (slightly in disbelief at this stage): I was expecting it more around the age 50-60 like the generations before me in my family, not 33...

Cue me being teary (which is rare for me)

THE WEEKS WENT BY AND IN MANY WAYS LIFE TOOK ON A NORMALITY AGAIN. WE ARRANGED FOR THE HICKMAN LINE TO BE FLUSHED AT HOME SO, ALTHOUGH THERE WERE STILL OCCASIONAL ISSUES WITH VISITS, THAT SEEMED TO RESOLVE HELGA'S FRUSTRATION. NOT BEING ON TREATMENT MEANT HELGA STARTED TO LOOK AND FEEL REALLY WELL. SHE CONTINUED TO WORK FROM HOME AND HER CONFIDENCE RETURNED - SHE EVEN AGREED TO DO A CHARITY FASHION SHOW...

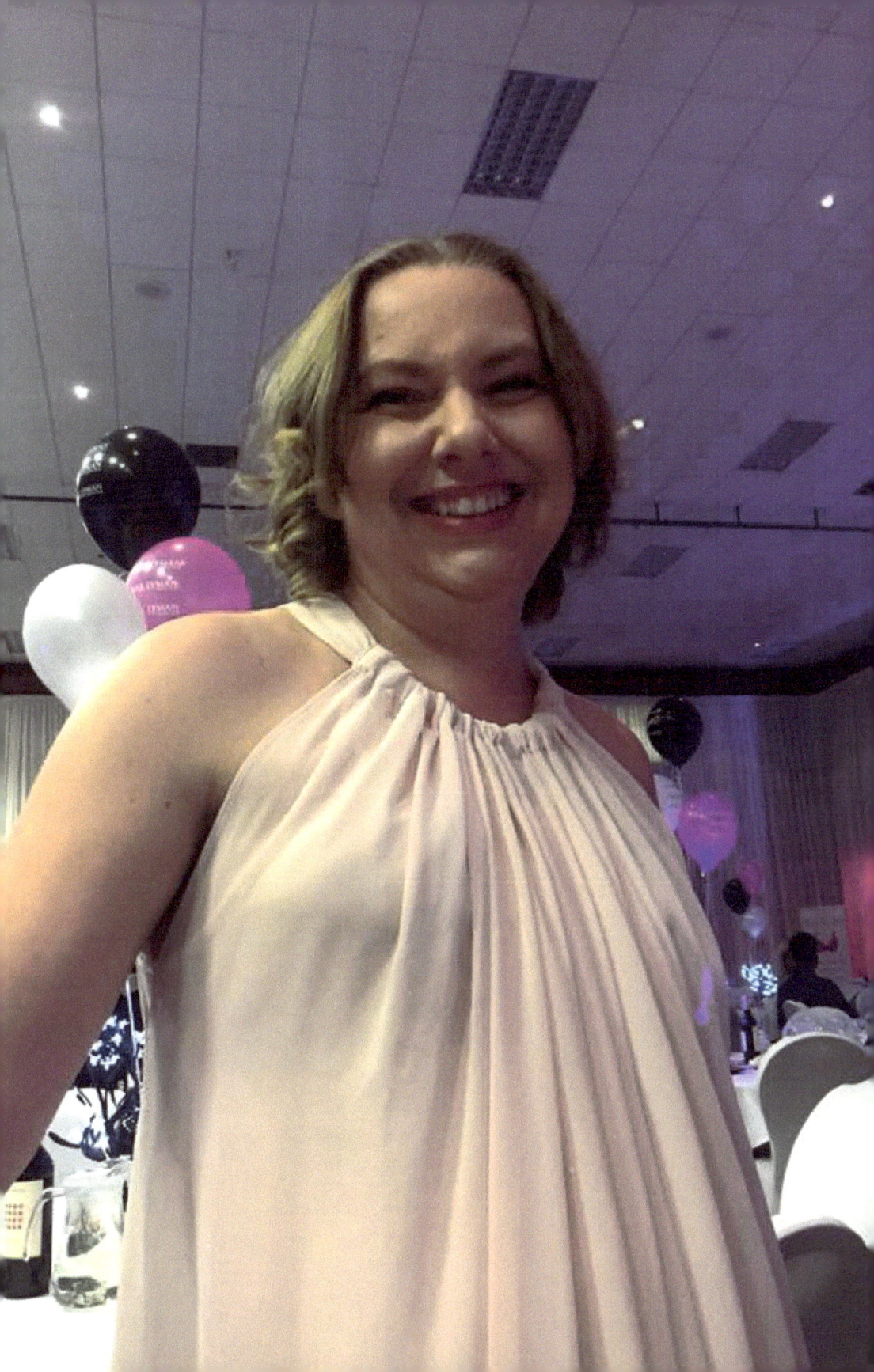

Helga Peeters
4th Sep 2018 at 23:06

I have done it - call me crazy...I've joined the 'completely bonkers' category...

Wednesday 24th October, yours truly is appearing in the Breast Cancer Fashion Show at The Chateau Impney about 6.30ish onwards.
£20 a ticket which includes a cheese platter and wine!

Who's up for cheering?!

😘

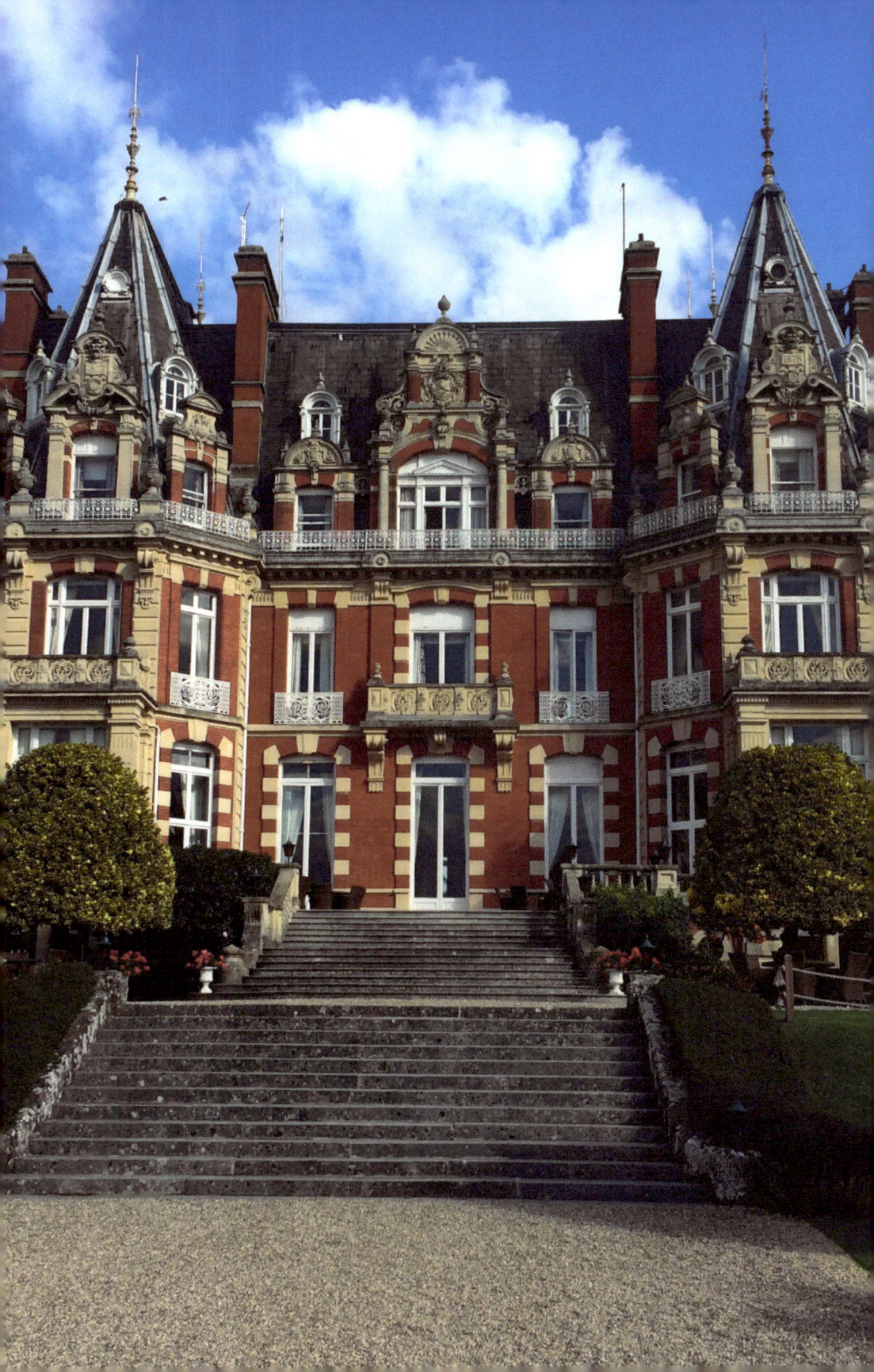

Helen Ainsley is with **Helga Peeters**
24th Oct 2018 at 21:55

Fantastic night at The Breast Cancer Charity Fashion Show!! Hats off to the lovely Helga who looked stunning in her posh frock and totally rocked the catwalk!!!

💕💕

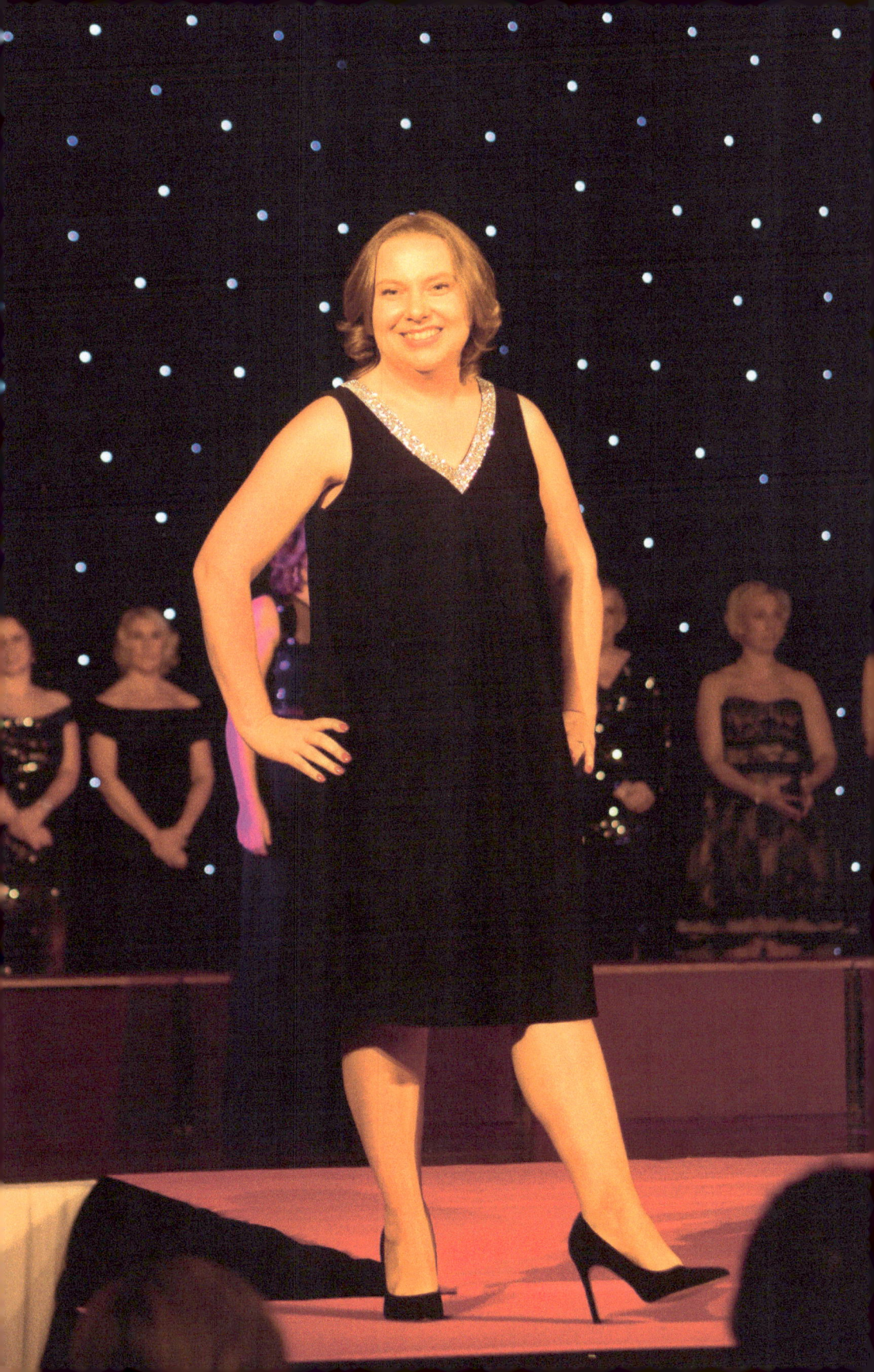

THEN, BEFORE WE KNEW IT, THE TIME HAD
COME TO SEE WHAT EFFECT 3 MONTHS
WITHOUT TREATMENT HAD HAD ON
THE CANCER...

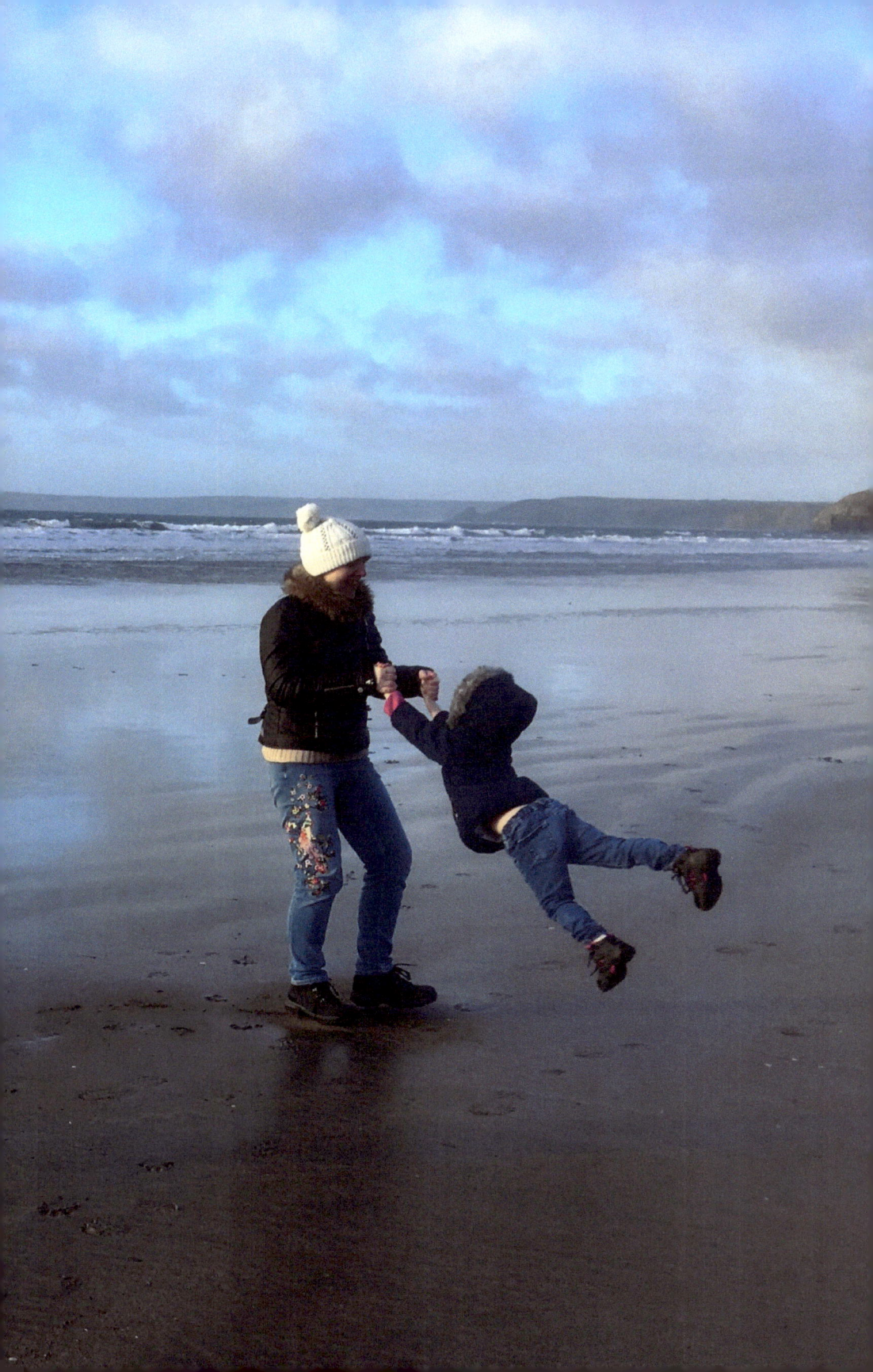

Helga Peeters is with **Justin Bowen**
10th Dec 2018 at 17:13

If people had asked me a few weeks ago what I wanted for Christmas, it would have been to hear we're stable and therefore got another 3 months off all treatments. It really has been lovely not feeling pants!

We had my 3-monthly scan at the end of November and had to go today for the results. If I'm honest, can't say it was something I was looking forward to particularly, but needs must and all. So, what was the outcome? I wish I had good news for you all, I really do. However it was inevitable with an aggressive form of metastatic breast cancer that with 3 months no treatment it would come back and bite me.

There's progression in my abdomen lymph glands, and a few nodes have now also been affected. Somehow miraculously I still have no symptoms (we've seen that before earlier in the year!).

As a result, next week I'm starting on Capecitabine for however long it works, every 3 weeks. Some side effects have been flagged up; the usual, with a few delightful ones Justin really is looking forward to, let me tell you! Anyway, rinse and repeat. At the end of the day, it is what it is and we can't do anything about it (gutted is more my feeling rather than being upset.)

Fingers crossed it works again, even if it's temporary like the others. There may be 1 or 2 more options after this and we have to look at trials out there... how long is a piece of string eh? My young age is definitely a downside as my cell multiplication goes way faster than people who are older.

C'est la vie. We keep playing whack-a-mole for as long as we can but it better not tamper with our Xmas dinner at Felice's this year! There would definitely be a fist-shake if I can't have my lobster ravioli!!!

🍽️ 🤣
Just keep swimming people 😘

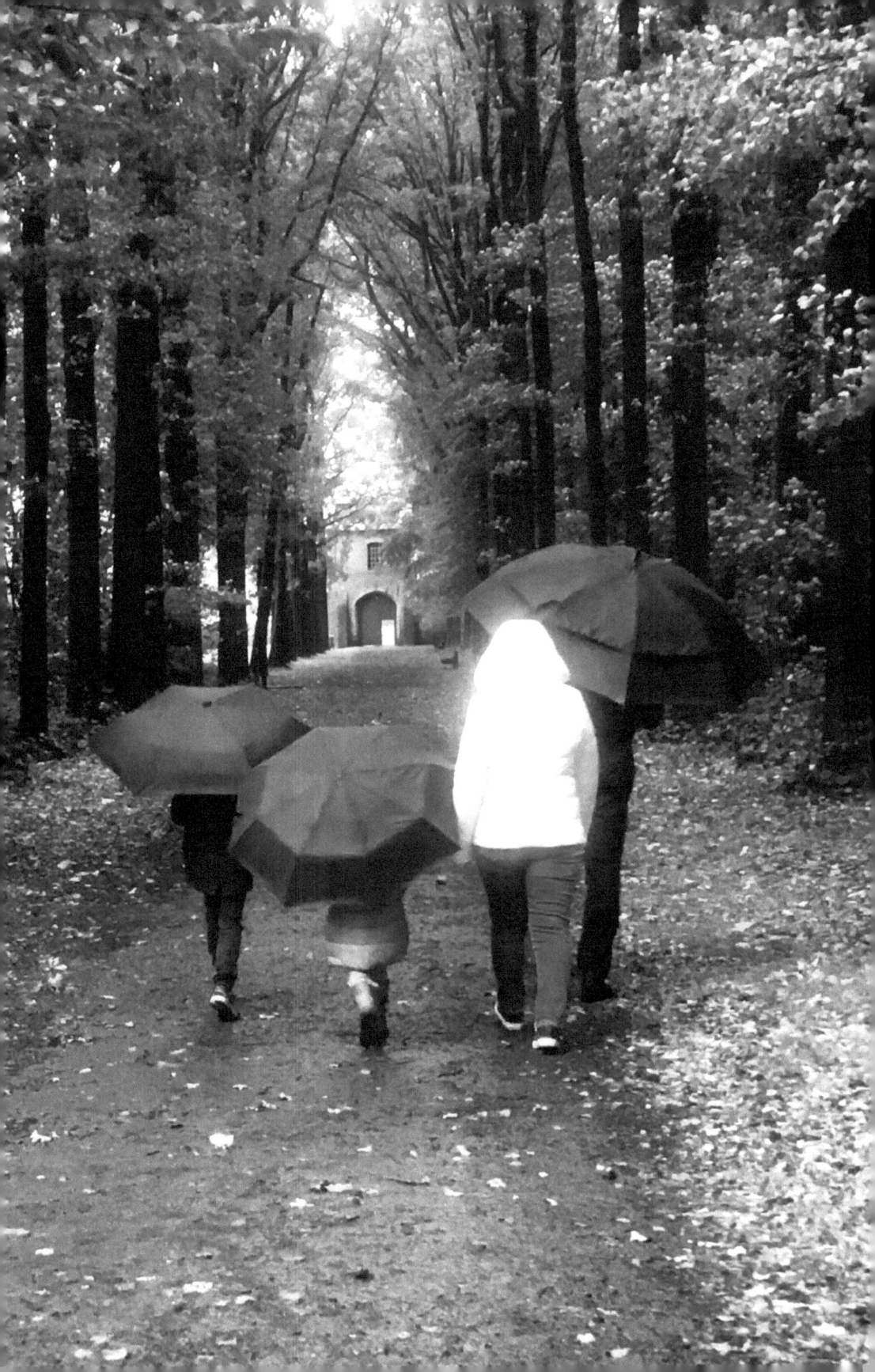

SO HERE'S THE THING. YOU GET THE FIRST
DIAGNOSIS. THAT'S A SHOCK. THEN YOU STEEL
YOURSELVES TO DO THE TREATMENT, TO GET
THROUGH IT, TO COME OUT THE OTHER SIDE.
YOU DO THAT. THEN THE NEXT BLOW COMES,
THE BRAIN TUMOURS. WHAT DO YOU DO? THE
SAME AGAIN. YOU GET THROUGH THAT. THEN
LIFE IS GOOD, NORMAL FOR A WHILE. YOU KNOW
THERE WILL BE A RECKONING AT SOME POINT
BECAUSE INSIDE HELGA'S BODY THE CANCER IS
STILL THERE, BUT YOU MILK THOSE TREATMENT-
FREE DAYS FOR ALL THEY'RE WORTH. THEN
YOU FIND OUT - THE CANCER HAS ALSO BEEN
MILKING THE TREATMENT-FREE DAYS. SO THEN
WHAT DO YOU DO?

WELL, WE WERE GETTING GOOD AT THIS. WE
WOULD GIVE OURSELVES 2 DAYS OF GRIEVING
(WHICH IS BASICALLY WHAT IT IS WHEN THE
GOOD LIFE YOU WERE LIVING COMES TO AN
END), THEN WE WOULD DO WHAT WE DO. WE
WOULD WORK ON THE BASIS THAT THE NEW
TREATMENT WOULD WORK AND MAKE DAMN
SURE WE KEPT OUR HOME AS POSITIVE AND
HAPPY AS WE POSSIBLY COULD.

BESIDES, A NEW YEAR WAS COMING, A CHANCE
TO FRESHEN OUR RESOLVE AND START AGAIN.

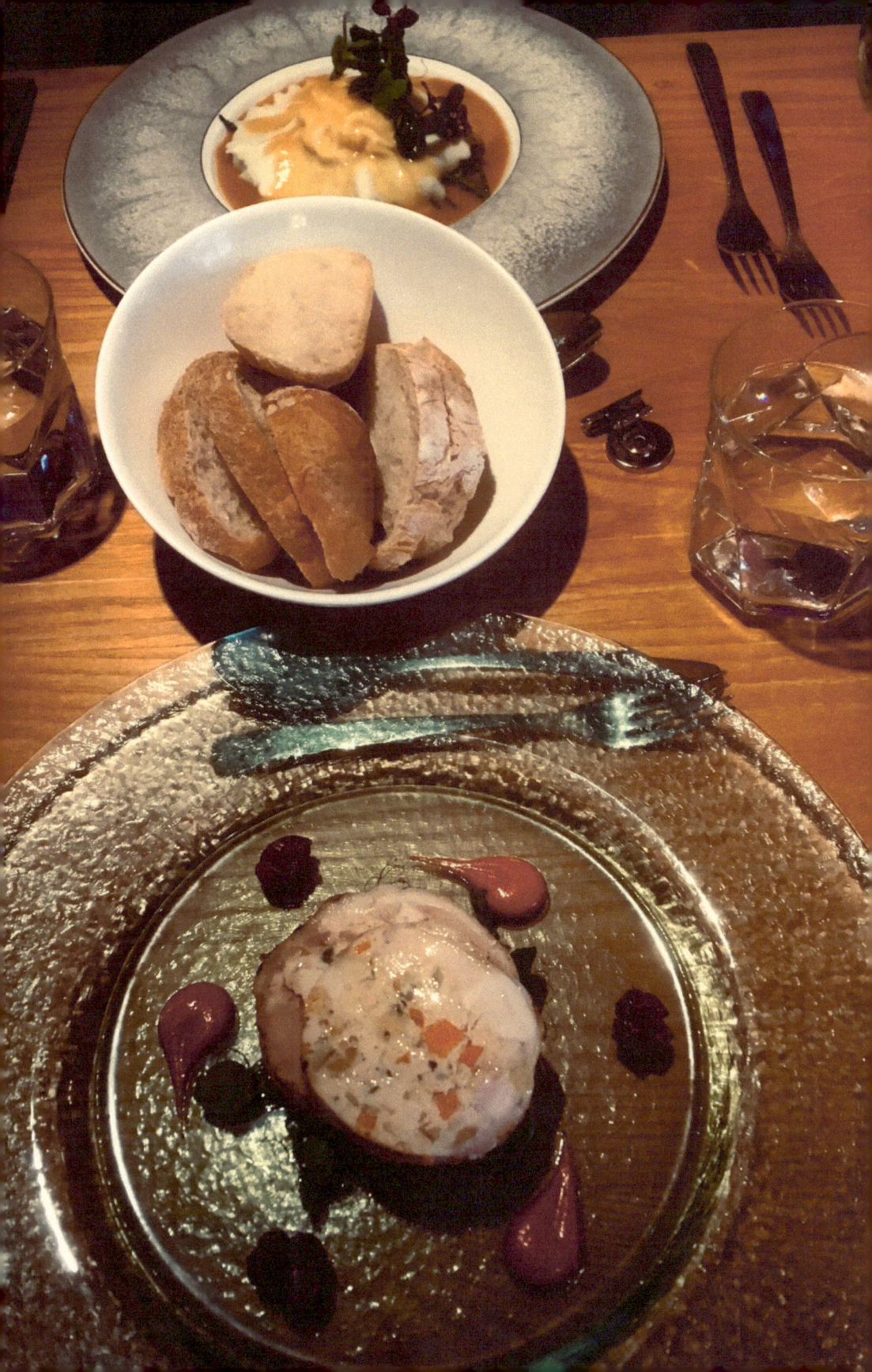

Helga Peeters
1st Jan 2019 at 17:13

Happy New Year everyone! 🥂
May you all have a good one

2018 can do one and be stuck with 2016 and 2017 where the sun doesn't shine. 3rd time lucky didn't work, so how about rainbow and sunshine after rain?

I don't do New Year's resolutions, but I'll go for I'll see you all in 2020? Just keep shining and be my light every day and I'll try to wear this body down and into the ground.

💕

Much love to you all xx

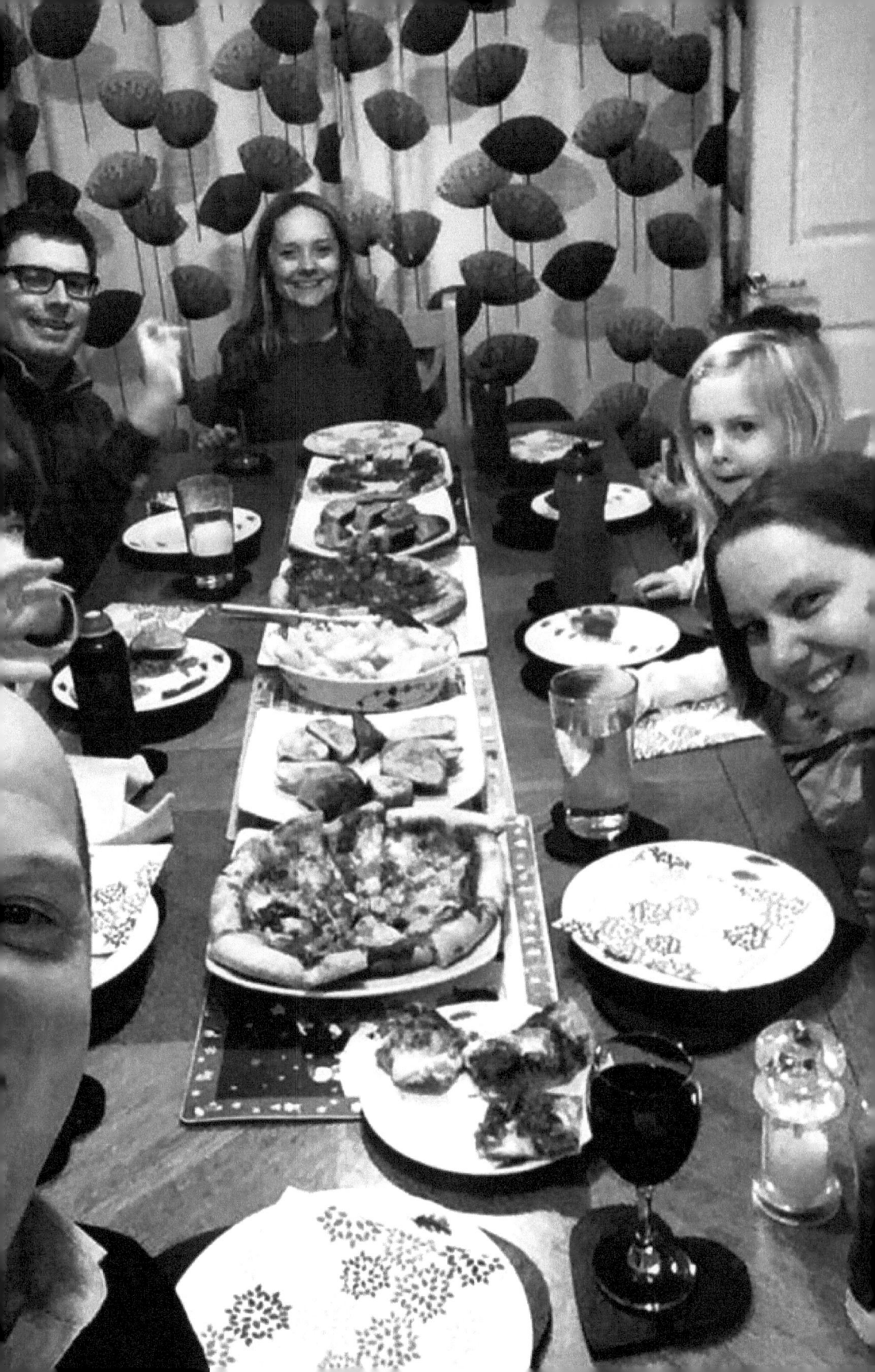

SO ON WE WENT. THANKFULLY,
CAPECITABINE PROVED TO BE RELATIVELY
MILD IN TERMS OF SIDE-EFFECTS WHICH
MEANT HELGA CONTINUED TO FEEL WELL
AND WAS ABLE TO DO PRETTY MUCH
EVERYTHING SHE WANTED TO DO (APART
FROM DRIVE!).

BACK IN THE NOW FAMILIAR ROUTINE OF
TREATMENT CYCLES, LIFE WAS STILL GOOD.

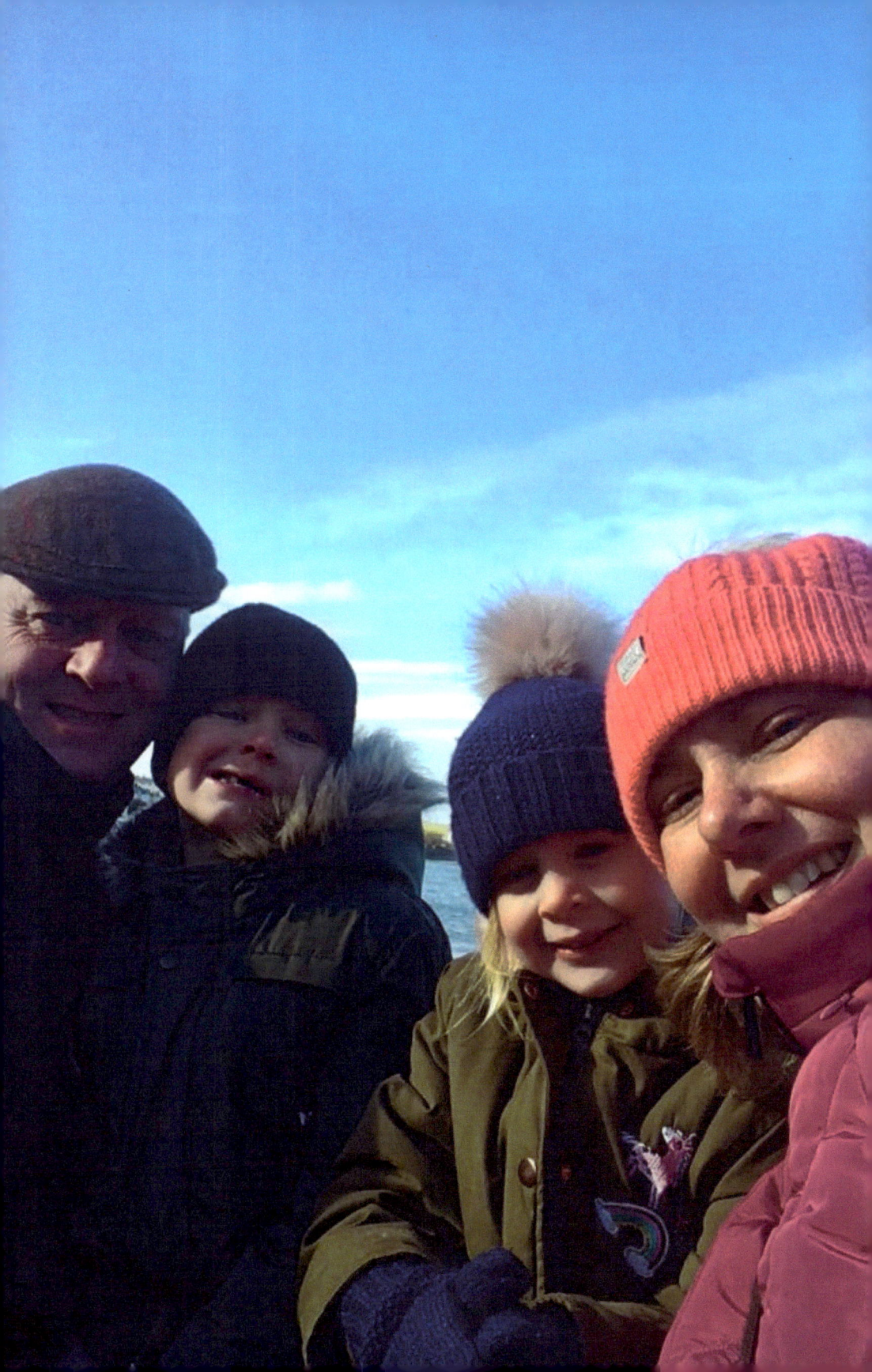

Helga Peeters
4th Feb 2019 at 07:35

Ah, apparently it's **'World Cancer Day'**

I can only look at it with mixed feelings. It's brought 2 extremes to life. One of days filled with happiness as I don't think I ever would have looked at life and enjoyed it as it is. It has also brought me the dark days of uncertainty.

I'll never be a fighter/survivor or any of that stuff. It will eventually claim me. I am merely doing what anyone in my shoes would be doing, and that's holding out as long as I can for my family and friends. But most of all for my 2 children who I wouldn't want to grow up without a mother. I am merely at the mercy of the medical world. They are the masters of this show.

Hoping one day something sticks or there will be a cure for my case. I can live and dream.

😉

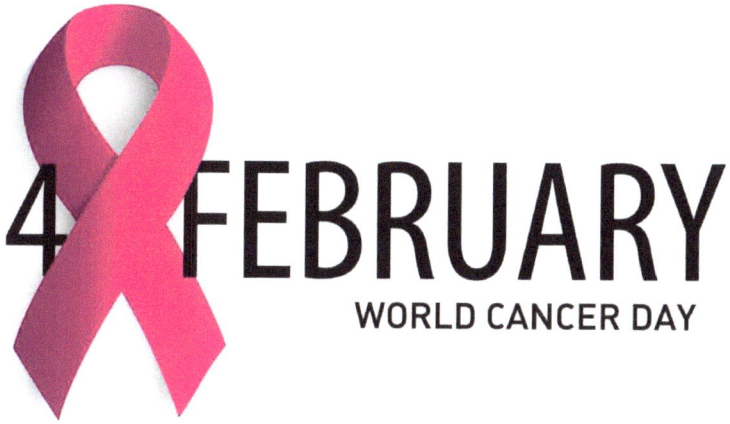

4 FEBRUARY

WORLD CANCER DAY

Helga Peeters
20th Feb 2019 at 13:56

Define a 'good mum.'

After all we are all trying our best and make mistakes along the way. There never is a parent manual and for those that are out there...get with it and get real.

However must be doing something right when after getting Seren out of the shower and wrapping her up yesterday, she says: "You're a good mummy". "Awww" I hear you go. So I asked her why she said that and she replied: " Because you look after us so well".

Bless her. Guess I'm doing something right somewhere.

👌 💗

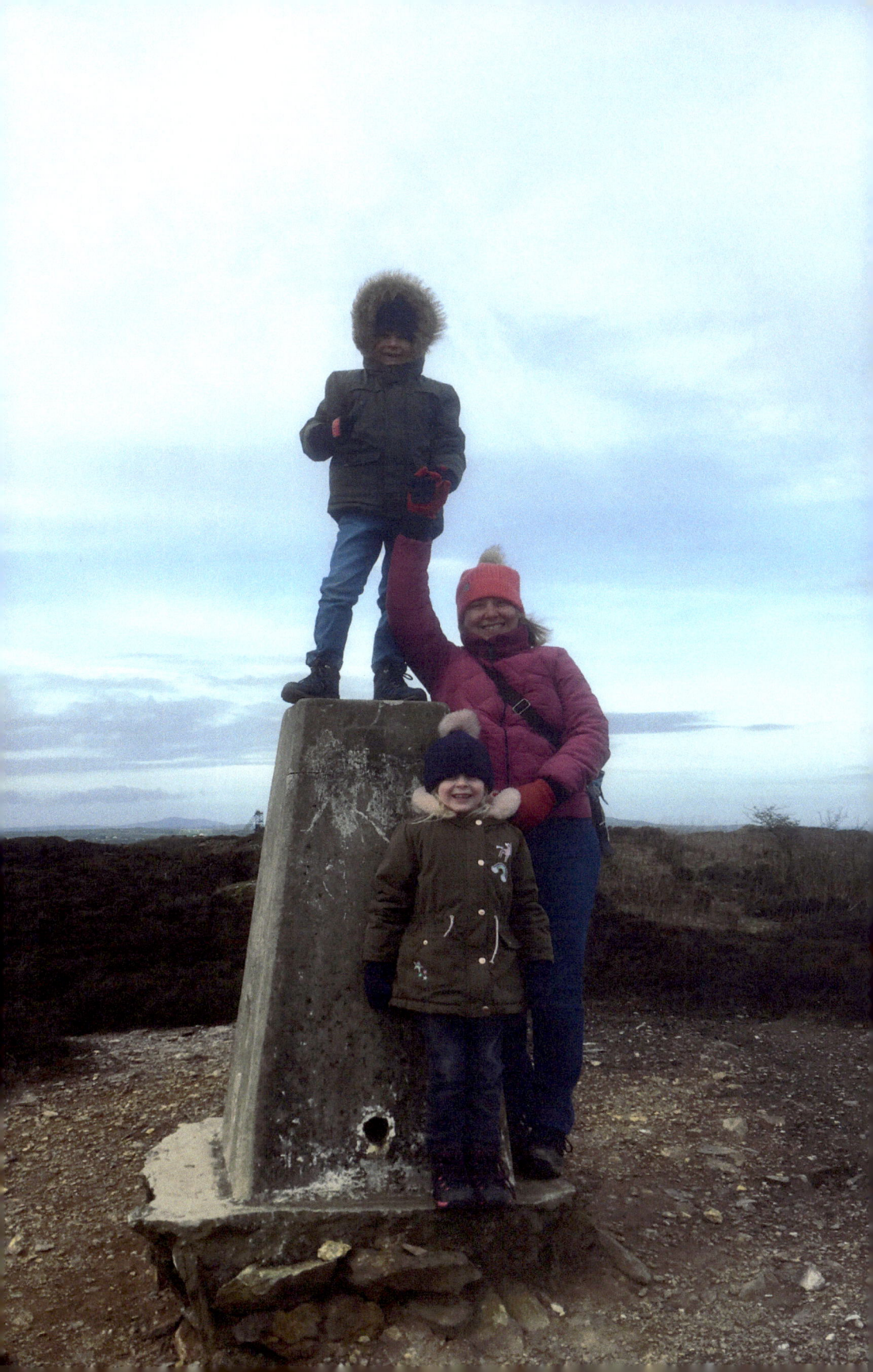

AFTER 3 MONTHS, YES YOU'VE GUESSED IT - SCAN, APPOINTMENT, RESULTS...

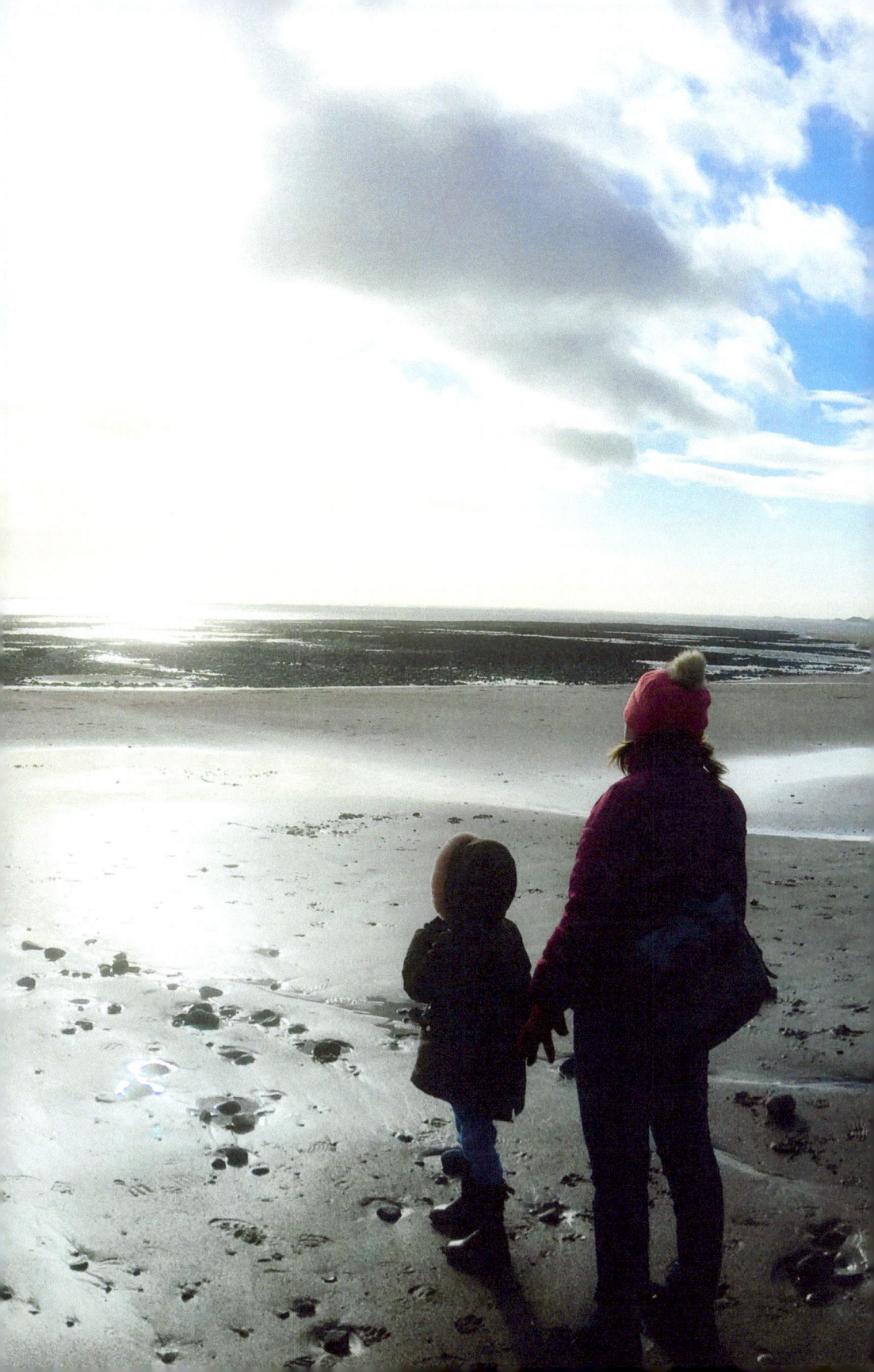

Justin Bowen is 🎉 celebrating this day with **Helga Peeters**
12th April 2019 at 17:15

Time for a pint after getting the news that Helga's chemo is working again and the tumours are on the retreat.

One thing we've learned is to make the most of days like this.

❤️

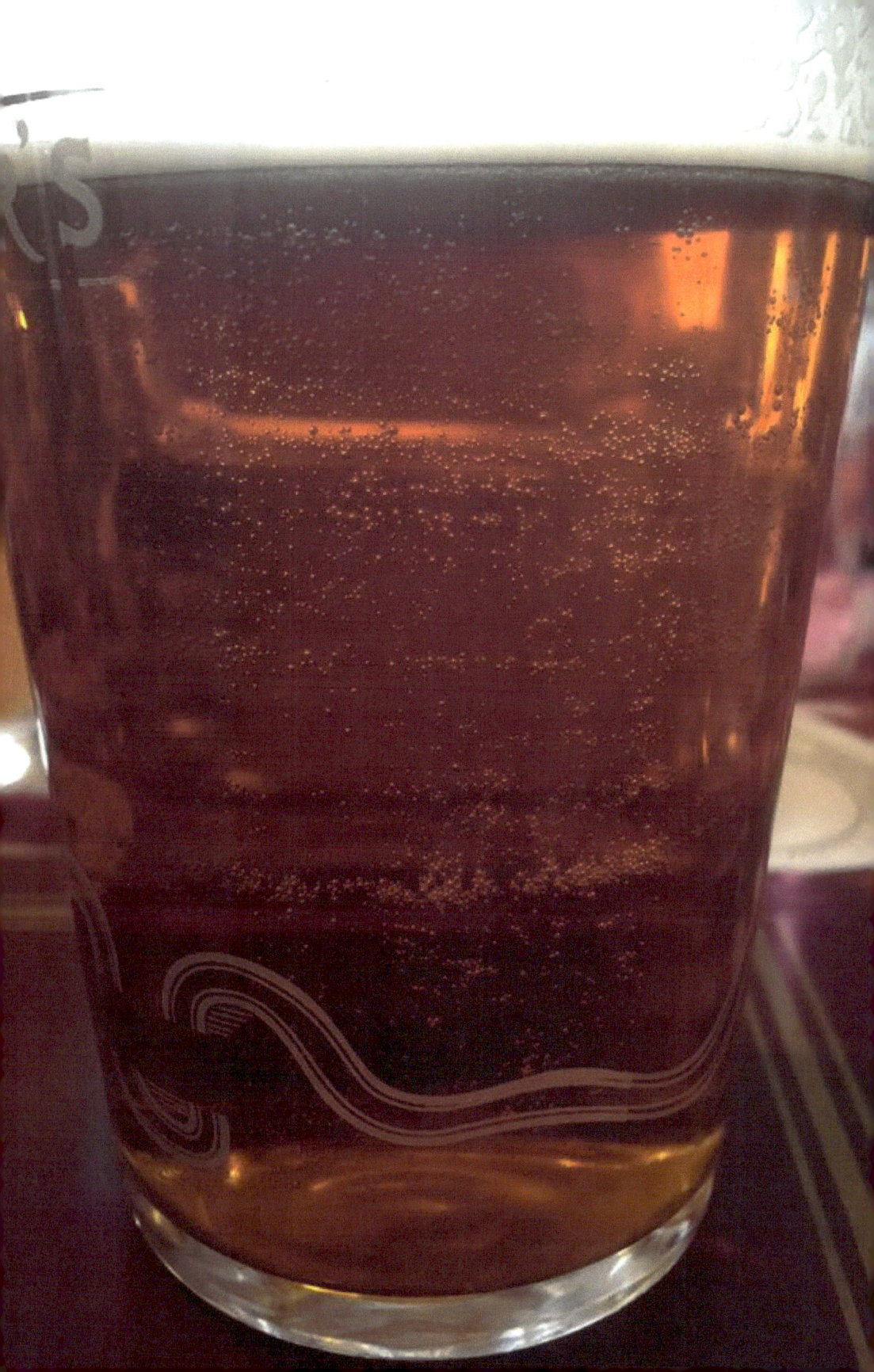

CAPECITABINE WAS PROVING EFFECTIVE
AT REDUCING THE TUMOURS IN HELGA'S
ABDOMEN AND TREATMENT CONTINUED.
ALTHOUGH THE DRUG WAS LIGHT IN SIDE-
EFFECTS, HELGA WAS FEELING LOW ON
ENERGY AND STRUGGLING TO BE AS ACTIVE
AS SHE WANTED TO BE.

Helga Peeters is 🙁 feeling frustrated
10th June 2019 at 21:18

It is hard sometimes to admit to yourself you are but a fraction of your former self at the age of 36.

I used to love Zumba, and though my legs still wanted to participate, the heart and particularly my right arm could not keep up.

I was like the 70-ish year old lady next to me. Struggling to follow like the others so we did our own thing.

It is frustrating sometimes certain things are now from an era I won't get back - might improve a bit but the lymphoedema risk isn't worth taking.

I think I'll stick to Yoga/Pilates and the odd bike ride and just have to accept my body is now like a 70-80 year old.

Pass me the gin...

ONE THING HELGA HAD BEEN AIMING
FOR EVER SINCE SHE'D BEEN DIAGNOSED
WITH BRAIN TUMOURS IN 2017 WAS TO BE
ALLOWED TO DRIVE AGAIN. THAT WOULD
ONLY HAPPEN ONCE THE TUMOURS HAD
BEEN STABLE FOR AT LEAST 12 MONTHS.

IN JUNE 2019 SHE HAD A SCAN ON HER
BRAIN TO SEE HOW THE TUMOURS WERE
DOING, SOME 2 YEARS AFTER BEING FIRST
DIAGNOSED WITH THEM.

THEN, ON 4TH JULY SHE WENT BACK TO SEE
HER CONSULTANT...

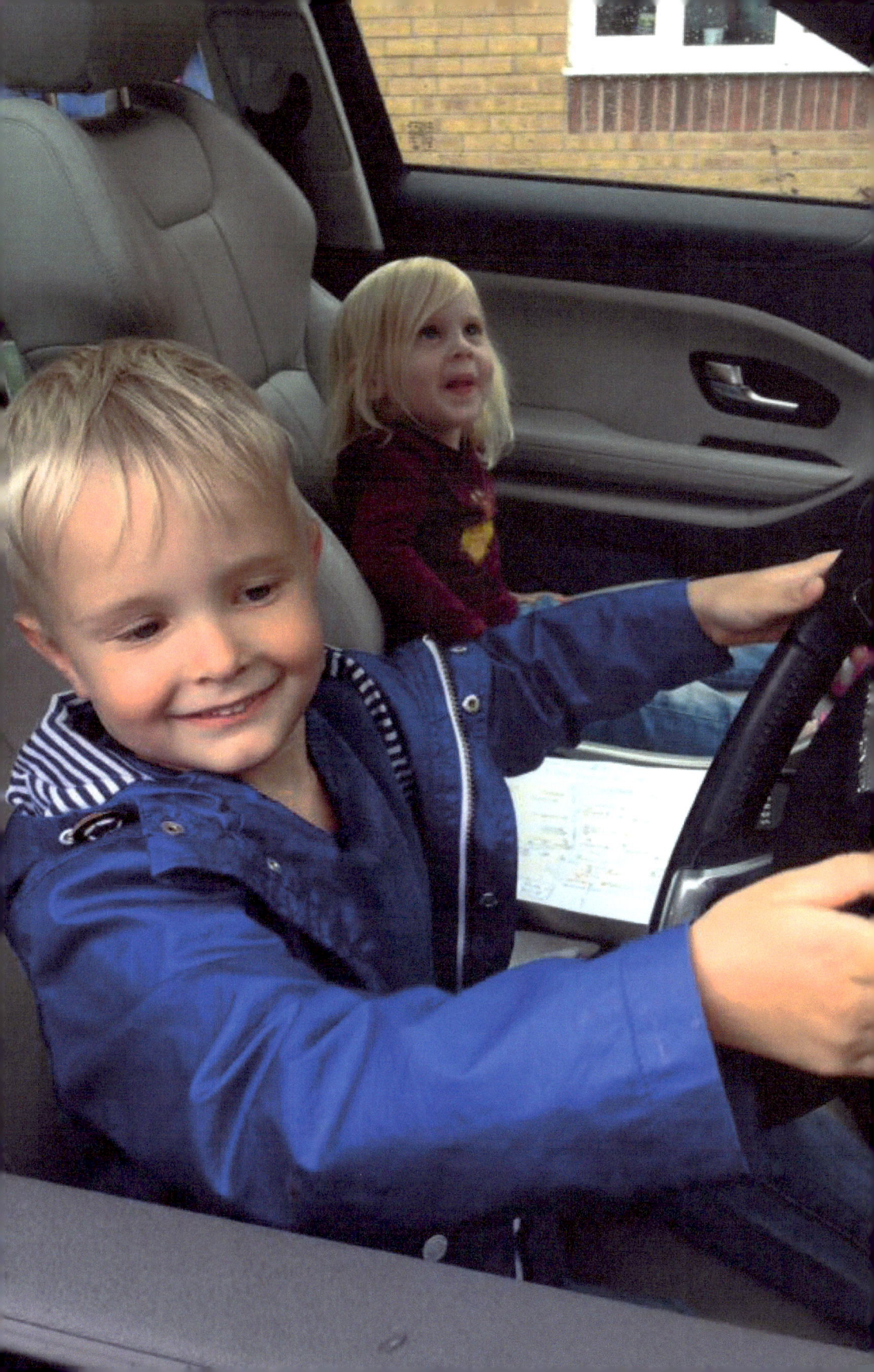

Justin Bowen
4th July 2019 at 16:06

Just over two years ago, after Helga's breast cancer spread to her brain, she was medically banned from driving. Today her wonderful NHS consultant, Dr Meade from The Queen Elizabeth Hospital, Birmingham (pictured) gave Helga the news that her tumours were stable enough for her to resume driving. We'll definitely be celebrating this!

❤️

#milestonemoment #newcartime #thankyounhs

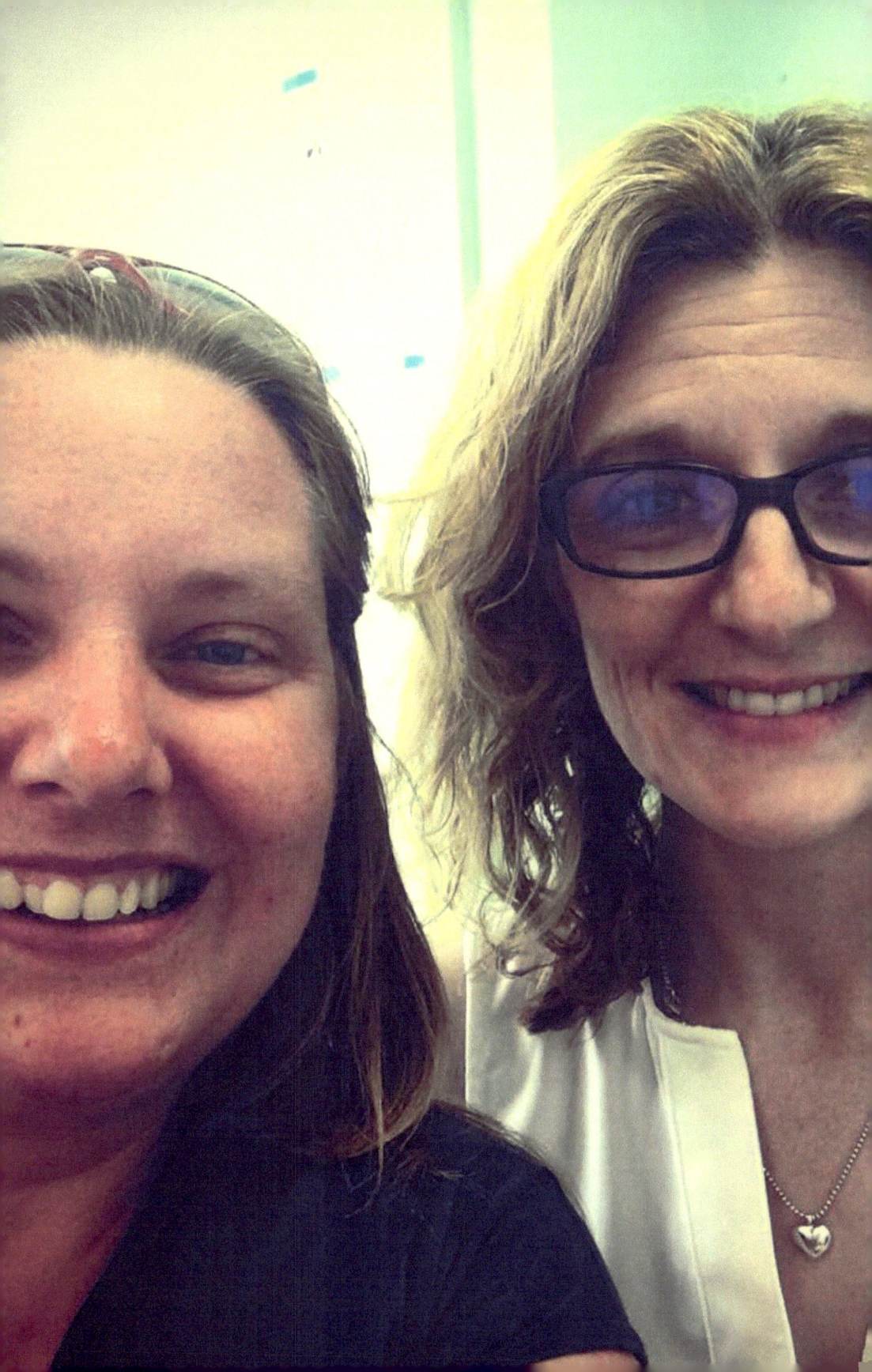

WITH A HOLIDAY TO RHODES BOOKED FOR THE END OF JULY, THIS WAS THE PERFECT NEWS. HELGA HAD BEEN PONDERING WHICH CAR SHE WAS GOING TO GET IF THE NEWS WAS GOOD, SO THERE WAS GREAT EXCITEMENT IN THE HOUSE ABOUT WHAT SHE WOULD CHOOSE. AN AUDI WAS LOOKING FAVOURITE!

THE NEXT MORNING, HELGA HAD A SCAN ON HER ABDOMEN TO MAKE SURE THE TUMOURS THERE WERE ALSO STILL UNDER CONTROL. HELGA HAD BEEN FEELING QUITE BLOATED IN HER BELLY, BUT WE HAD NO PARTICULAR CONCERNS.

THAT AFTERNOON, ON THE WAY TO PICK THE CHILDEN UP FROM SCHOOL, HELGA RECEIVED A PHONE CALL...

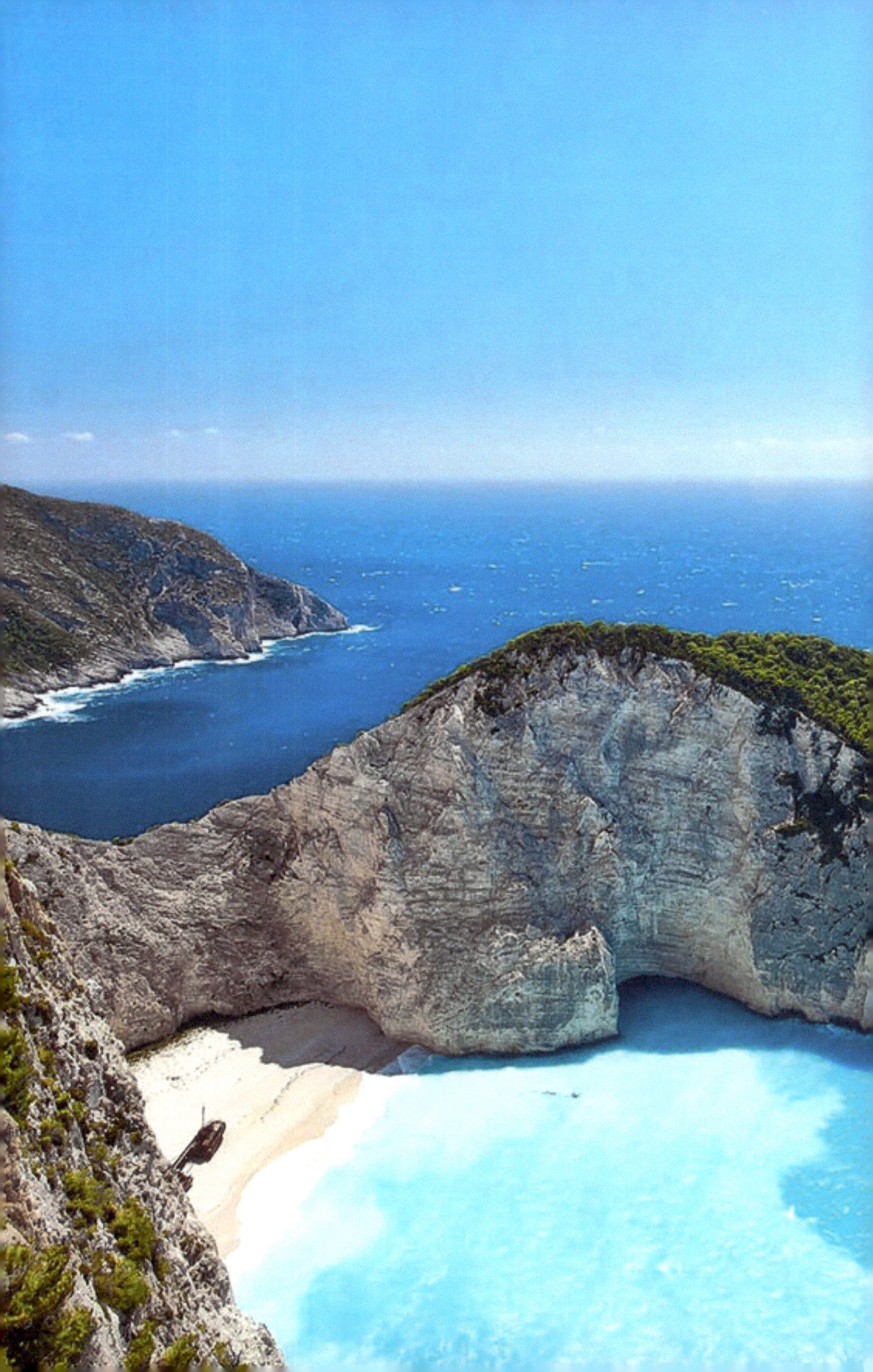

Helga Peeters is 🙁 feeling frustrated
5th Jul 2019 at 18:03

Well, welcome everyone to the cancer rollercoaster. After my happy news yesterday, I got a phone call from the oncologist this afternoon after my scan to say there's a small blockage in my liver caused by cancer spread.

That's right people, here we are again. To say I'm slowly starting to have enough is an understatement.

What's next? Well, more tests, another tube being inserted to bypass the blockage and drain liver into my bowel. They said to go on holiday in 2 weeks but before/after is going to be quite busy again until a new plan has been worked out based on the results of all the tests.

Happy Friday everyone! If I could tolerate it I'd be having a large friggin beverage.

🙄

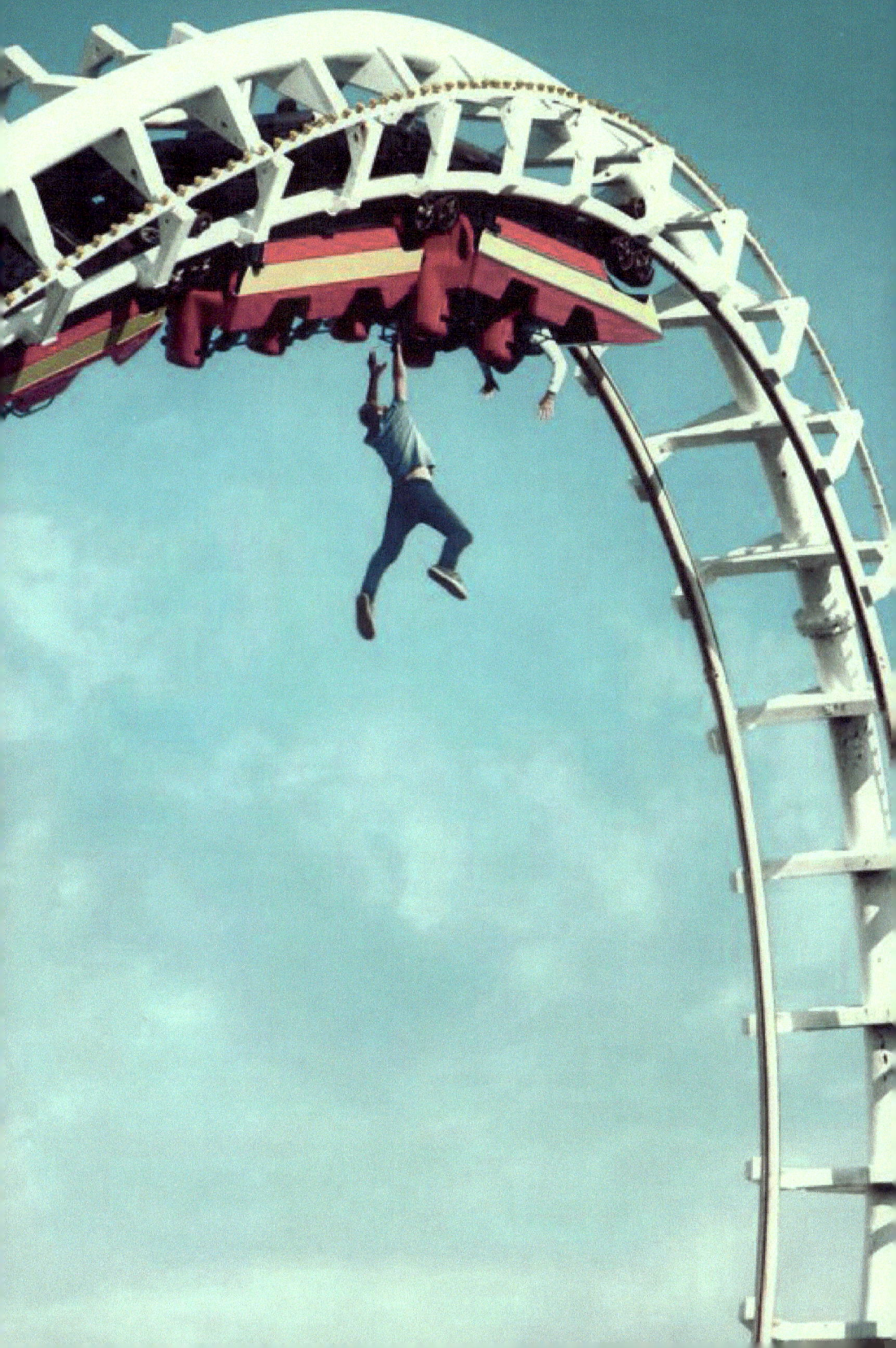

SO, AFTER WHAT SEEMED LIKE JUST A FEW
SHORT MONTHS, CAPECITABINE HAD
STOPPED WORKING. THE CANCER HAD
SPREAD TO HELGA'S LIVER, WHICH WAS
CAUSING A BLOCKAGE AND MAKING HER
BELLY SWELL WITH FLUID.

WE HAD ALWAYS KEPT THE CHILDREN
FULLY INFORMED ABOUT HELGA'S CANCER
AND THE TREATMENTS SHE WAS HAVING.
WE ALWAYS ANSWERED THEIR QUESTIONS
HONESTLY. OVER THE NEXT FEW DAYS,
HELGA'S BELLY BECAME VERY SWOLLEN
AND THE CHILDREN QUICKLY NOTICED. SO
WE EXPLAINED TO THEM WHY, AND THAT
"MUMMY WILL BE STARTING A NEW
MEDICINE SOON."

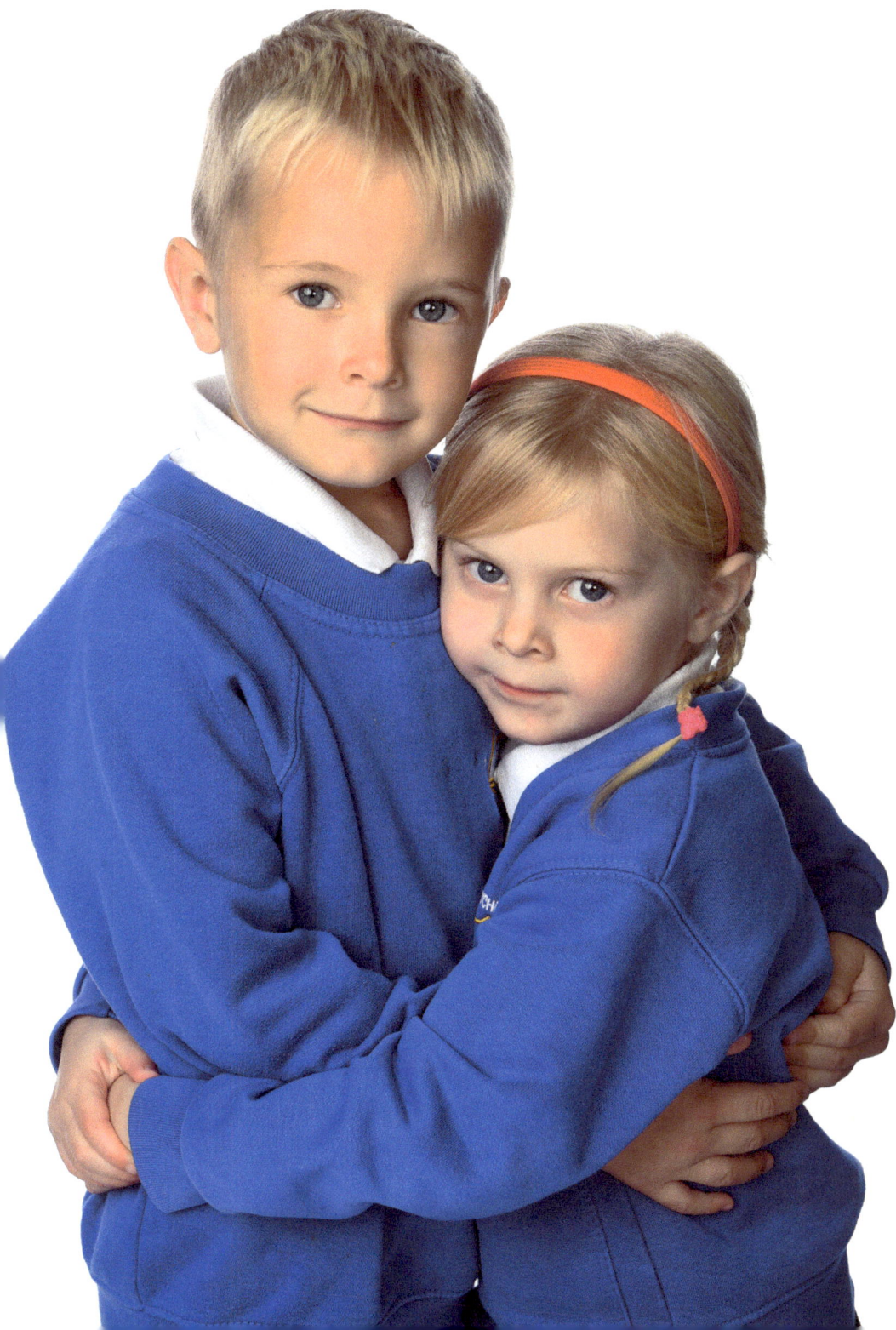

Justin Bowen is 😌 feeling thoughtful with **Helga Peeters**
10th Jul 2019 at 20:56

What do you tell a 7 year old who realises his mum isn't well? Now that Helga's cancer has spread to her liver it's made her belly very bloated. Tonight the little man said that if the doctors can't fix 'Mummy's belly' she'll die, and he's really worried about that. I told him "Well, they fixed the lump in her breast, and they fixed the lump when it was on her brain and I think they'll fix it now it's making her belly very bloated, so right now I'm not worried. But it's ok that you are worried and I understand that you are, so what I promise is that although at this moment I think Mummy will be here until she's old and wrinkled and talks with a croaky voice, if anything changes I'll let you know."

He seemed happy with that, but f**k me this s**t is hard sometimes.

🤹

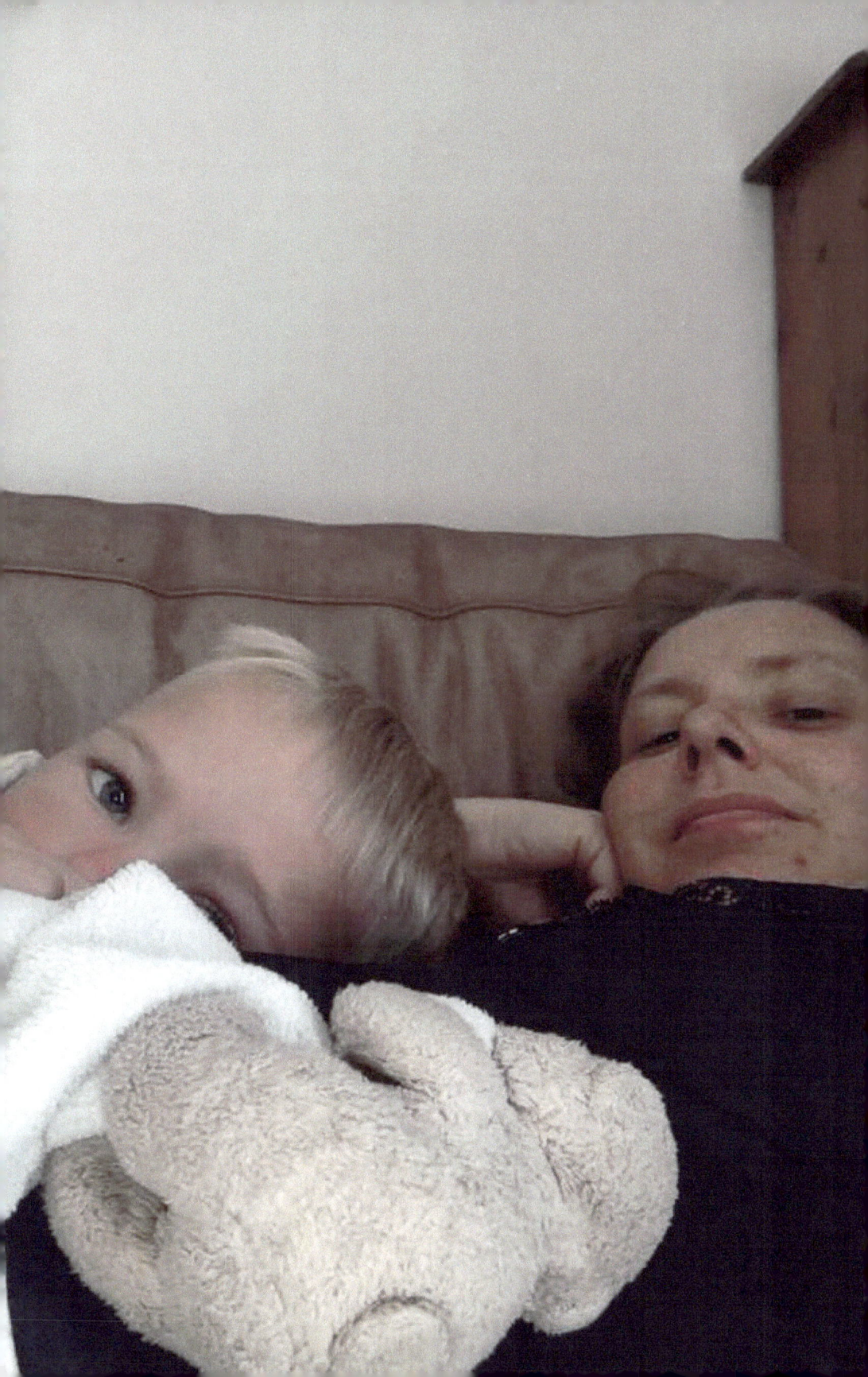

OUR HOLIDAY, WHICH WAS BOOKED FOR
SUNDAY JULY 21ST, WAS NOW A LITTLE OVER
A WEEK AWAY. HELGA'S BELLY HAD BECOME
SO SWOLLEN SHE WAS STRUGGLING TO EAT.
IT HAD TO BE DRAINED OR SHE WOULDN'T
BE WELL ENOUGH TO TRAVEL. SHE WAS
ADMITTED TO HOSPITAL ON 16TH JULY.

Helga Peeters is at **Worcestershire Acute Hospitals NHS Trust**
16th Jul 2019 at 14:36 · Worcester, Worcestershire ·

Well, the girl out of Charlie and the Chocolate Factory is finally going to get juiced! Hopefully not for too long as they say depending on the amount of fluid it can take a day or up to a few days.

Christ get me to Rhodes!!!!

😟

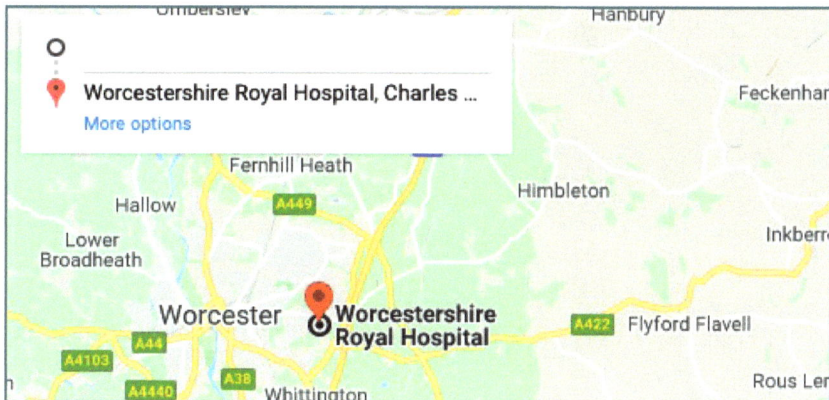

Helga Peeters
17th Jul 2019 at 15:22

Little update before I get millions of questions... 😉

They hooked me on today and within less than 1 hour nearly 4 litres came spouting out. Still hooked on at the moment but coming off soon as it has massively slowed down over the hours. I am now nearly on 5. 5-6 litres of fluid drained.

Imagine carrying that with you all the time! 😱

Anyways, eaten for the first time in a week - still not a lot, but much better so they were happy. Kidneys took a battering over the last few weeks though and were found to be dehydrated. So I'm receiving 2 bags to rehydrate kidneys again and if bloods come back ok, I could potentially go home tomorrow morning.

Feeling much better now I can breathe is all I'm saying. The pressure of that amount of fluid is now gone and I actually feel like I've got room again.

😬

Might actually get to go on holiday now. 🤞

HELGA RETURNED HOME FEELING MUCH BETTER AND WE COULD FINALLY LOOK FORWARD TO HAVING OUR HOLIDAY.

HOWEVER, BEFORE THAT WE HAD ONE LAST APPOINTMENT WITH THE ONCOLOGIST TO FIND OUT WHAT THE NEW TREATMENT WOULD BE. IT WAS BOOKED FOR FRIDAY 19TH JULY, 2 DAYS BEFORE WE WERE DUE TO GO ON HOLIDAY.

Justin Bowen is with **Helga Peeters**
19th Jul 2019 at 17:15

Hi all,

Earlier today we had Helga's latest appointment with her oncologist. Unfortunately the cancer is now in her liver (which we knew) and also her lungs. As the damage to her liver is significant, her body wouldn't be able to stand another round of chemotherapy which means that there's nothing else they can do to stop the disease growing. So it's likely that Helga has a matter of months to live now. The damage to her lungs also means that she won't be able to fly for our holiday. Your support for our family has been magnificent since Helga was first diagnosed and we feel very lucky to have such wonderful people around us as we face the weeks and months ahead.

Love to you all

Justin and Helga...

❤️

IT'S HARD TO DESCRIBE WHAT IT'S LIKE TO
HEAR THAT NO FURTHER TREATMENT IS
POSSIBLE. IT'S EVEN HARDER TO DESCRIBE
WHAT IT'S LIKE TELLING YOUR CHILDREN
THAT THERE IS NOTHING MORE THAT THE
DOCTORS CAN DO AND THAT THEIR MUM
WILL SOON DIE. BUT HOWEVER HARD IT ALL
IS, WE KNEW THAT IT WAS UP TO US TO MAKE
THE MOST OF EVERY SINGLE MOMENT OF
WHATEVER TIME WE HAD LEFT TOGETHER.

AS HELGA COULDN'T FLY, AND WE COULDN'T
GO ON OUR PLANNED HOLIDAY TO RHODES,
WE DECIDED TO HAVE A FEW DAYS HOLIDAY
IN NORFOLK. THIS INCLUDED GOING BACK
TO MUNDESLEY WHERE WE HAD SPENT
A DAY SHORTLY AFTER HELGA WAS FIRST
DIAGNOSED IN 2016.

FORTUNATELY THE SUN SHONE AS
TEMPERATURES REACHED 30 DEGREES FOR
A DAY ON ONE OF OUR FAVOURITE BEACHES
WITH THE CHILDREN AND THEIR COUSINS.
WE COULDN'T HAVE ASKED FOR A MORE
PERFECT DAY.

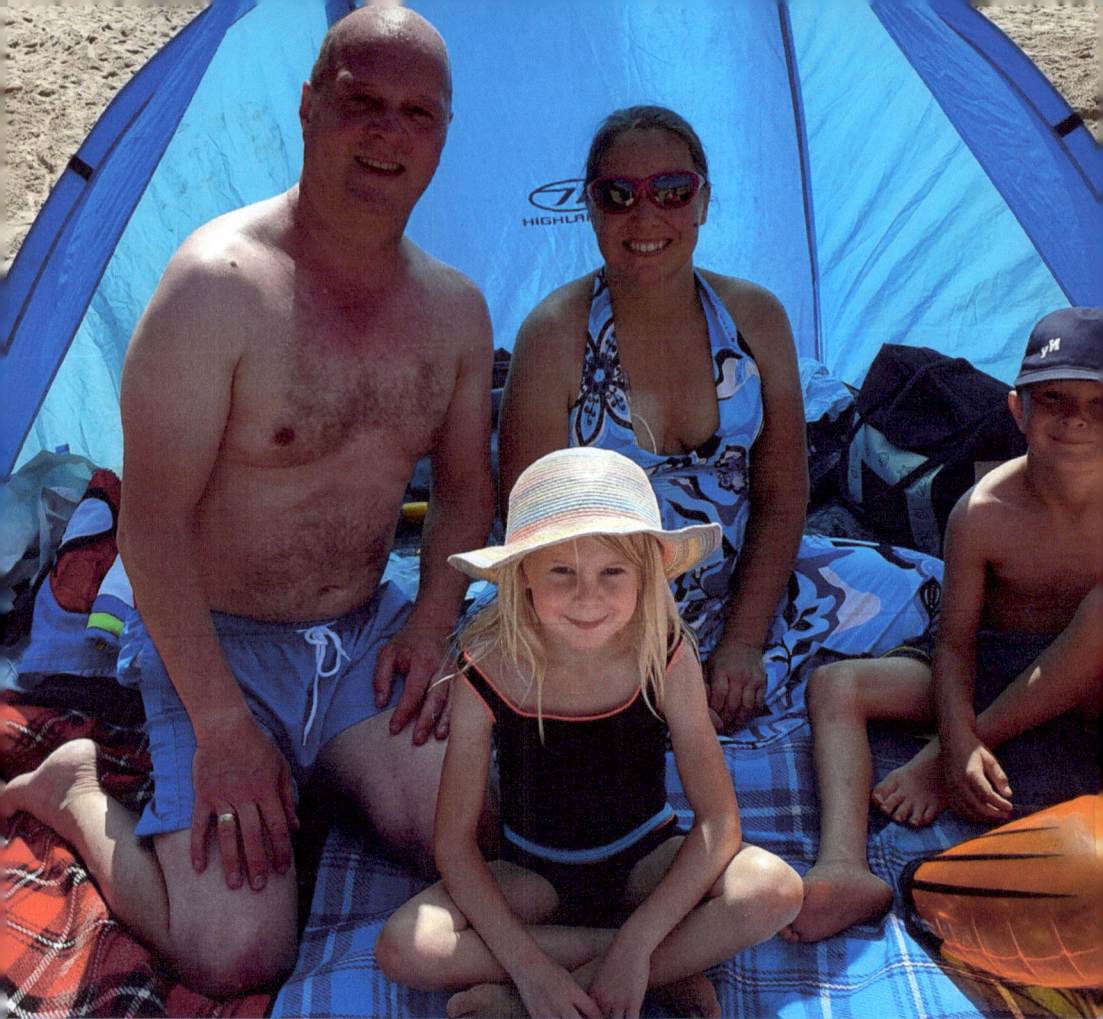
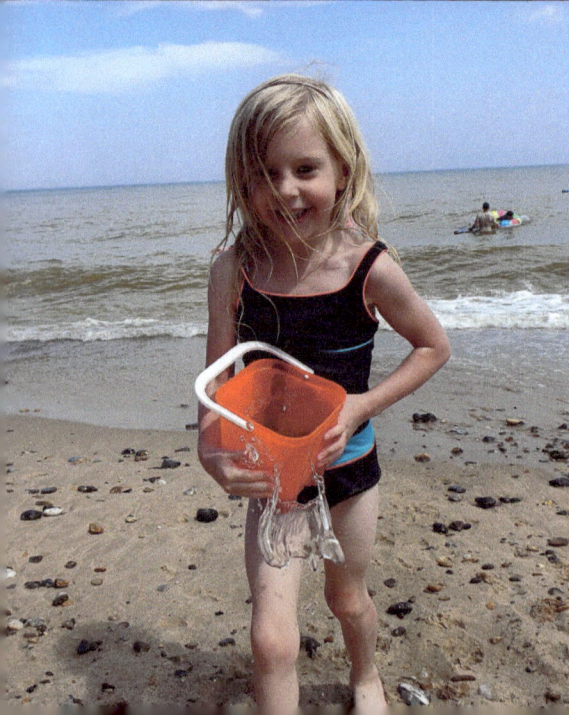
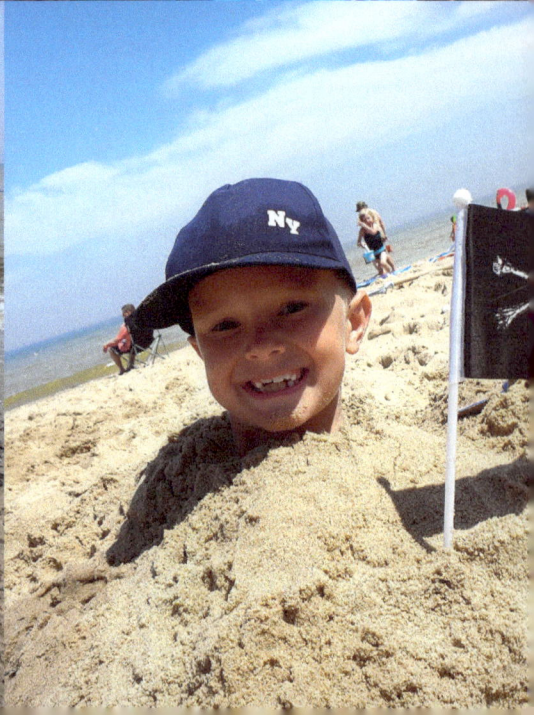

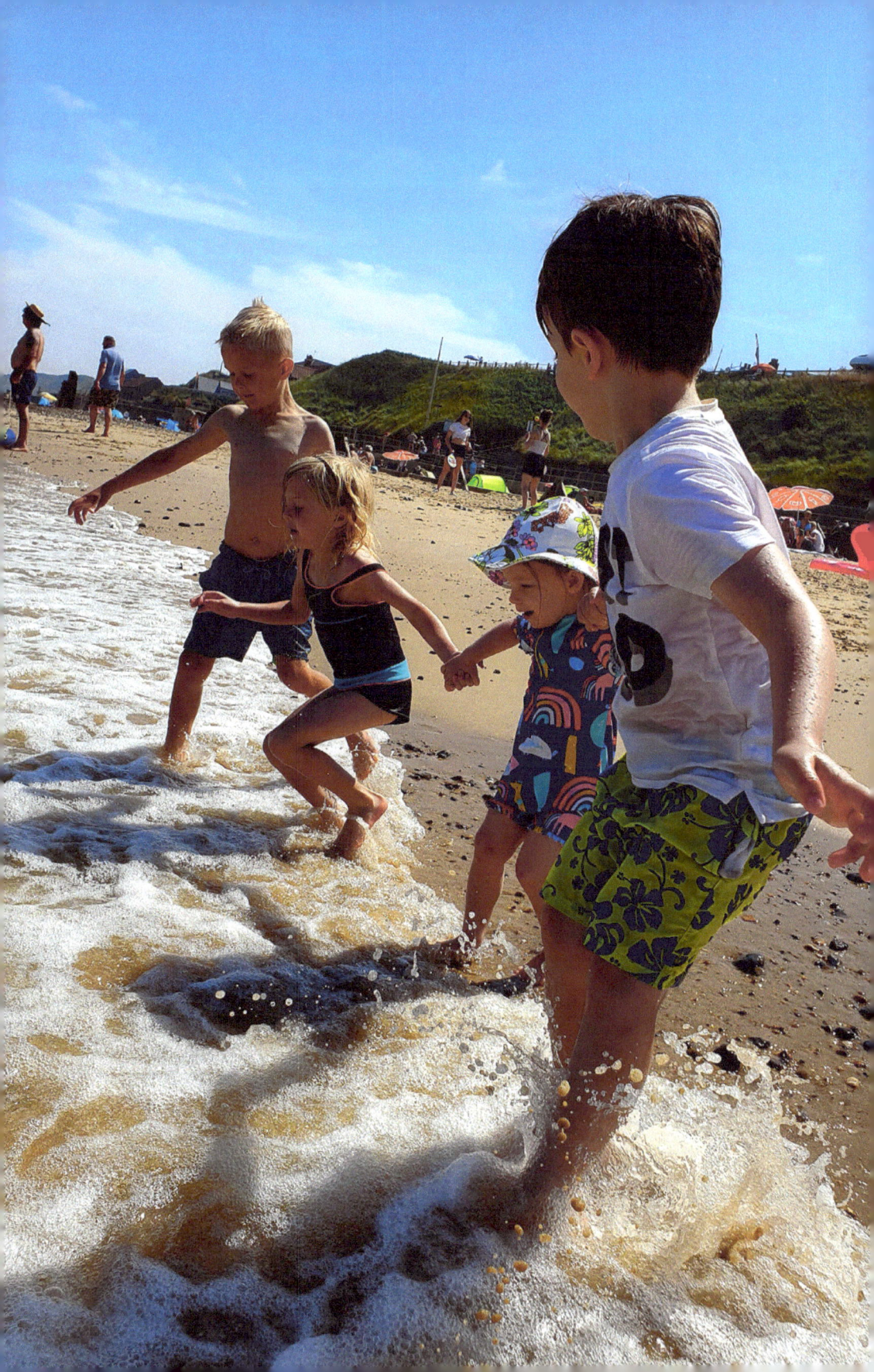

ON SATURDAY 27TH JULY, WE ROUNDED OFF OUR 'ALTERNATIVE HOLIDAY' WEEK WITH A DAY AT DRAYTON MANOR PARK. OVER THE COURSE OF THE DAY, HELGA STARTED TO FEEL UNWELL AND DEVELOPED A SLIGHT TEMPERATURE. BY 11.15PM, IT HAD RISEN TO 39 DEGREES. ALTHOUGH WE WEREN'T OVERLY CONCERNED, IT WAS HIGH ENOUGH FOR THE DOCTOR TO RECOMMEND HELGA BE ADMITTED TO HOSPITAL. WE THOUGHT SHE WOULD BE HOME WITHIN A COUPLE OF DAYS.

Justin Bowen is with **Helga Peeters** at
Worcestershire Acute Hospitals NHS Trust · Worcestershire
30th Jul 2019 at 20:07

Just an update for everyone on Helga's condition. Having been admitted to hospital on Saturday night with a Strep B infection, Helga is now on Silver Ward at Worcester Hospital. The infection had been dealt with but to prevent it coming back, she will have her Hickman line removed, which hopefully will happen tomorrow or Thursday. Additionally, her liver cancer means that her belly is getting bloated very quickly and needs urgently draining. After a bit of a battle today we've got Helga's first on the list to have this tomorrow. So all in all, hoping to have her home within 24-48 hours.

🤞

In the mean time, feel free to visit Helga on Silver Ward. There are restrictions on visiting times (just avoid 12-1pm and 5-6pm), with 10pm being the latest. Only 2 people at a time though.

With love and continued thanks for your support,

Justin

❤️

Justin Bowen is with **Helga Peeters** at
Worcestershire Acute Hospitals NHS Trust
2nd August 2019 at 11:11 · Worcester, Worcestershire ·

Hi everyone

Just a little update on Helga. She will be staying in hospital until at least tomorrow. This is because when the drain was fitted to her belly, the huge amount of fluid that was released caused a big drop in her blood pressure, making her very weak. So until her blood pressure recovers she'll need to stay in hospital.

If anyone wishes to visit, she is on Silver Ward and visiting times are 9am until 10pm, apart from meal times (12-1pm and 5-6pm).

IN THE HOURS THAT FOLLOWED, HELGA'S
CONDITION DETERIORATED RAPIDLY.
IT BECAME CLEAR THAT WITH NO
CHEMOTHERAPY TO KEEP THE CANCER
CONTAINED IT HAD RAPIDLY SPREAD
THROUGH HER BODY. HER BRAIN TUMOURS
HAD RETURNED WITH A VENGEANCE AND
HER ORGANS BEGAN TO FAIL. BY AUGUST 3RD
WE KNEW THAT HELGA WOULD SOON DIE.
SHE WOULDN'T BE COMING HOME.

Justin Bowen is with **Helga Peeters** at
Worcestershire Acute Hospitals NHS Trust
4th August 2019 at 15:35 · Worcester, Worcestershire ·

Hi everyone,

Thank you for your continued love and support for Helga. It's a source of great strength to me and the children.

Helga is still in hospital having been suffering from vomiting and dizziness this morning. It's thought this is because her brain tumours have now returned. She has been given steroids earlier to counteract the effects and we're waiting to see if they work. She's currently asleep so we won't know until later whether they've helped. If they are effective, Helga will have a day or two at home before going into a hospice. If they are not she will stay in hospital until she can move into a hospice. The situation is very fluid and so it's a question of waiting. Either way, I think it's fair to say we are probably looking at days, with a slim possibility of a couple of weeks left.

In terms of visiting, once it becomes clearer where Helga will be later I'll let everyone know.

Thank you again - you're all wonderful.

❤️

Justin Bowen is with **Helga Peeters**
5th August 2019 at 06:35

Good morning everyone

I've had alot of messages asking about visiting Helga. Sorry if I haven't managed to reply to you all, I thought it easier if I say it here.

The amount of love for Helga has been a defining feature of her life. Now at this time it really has been a great source of strength for me and the children too. So, if you want to come and say goodbye to Helga then please come - she doesn't have long left. Don't worry if I'm with her, just come. (Visiting times on Silver Ward are 9am to 10pm. If she moves to a hospice I will let you know)

Just remember there is a limit of 3 people by the bed, so you may have to wait outside the ward for a while - there may be a queue! Helga loves our English traditions, so if there is a nice, orderly queue of people waiting to see her it would be very fitting!

Love to you all

Justin

❤️

Justin Bowen is with **Helga Peeters**
6th August 2019 at 07:57

Good morning everyone

Last night, shortly after 8pm, my beautiful wife Helga passed away. She was surrounded by 5 wonderful people who loved her dearly and in the words of one of those present, she passed *"as lightly as a feather"*

I will miss her beyond words.

Thank you for all your love and support in particular to **Maddy, Lorna, Seb, Helena** and **Fran,** who were with her at the end.

You are all wonderful.

❤️

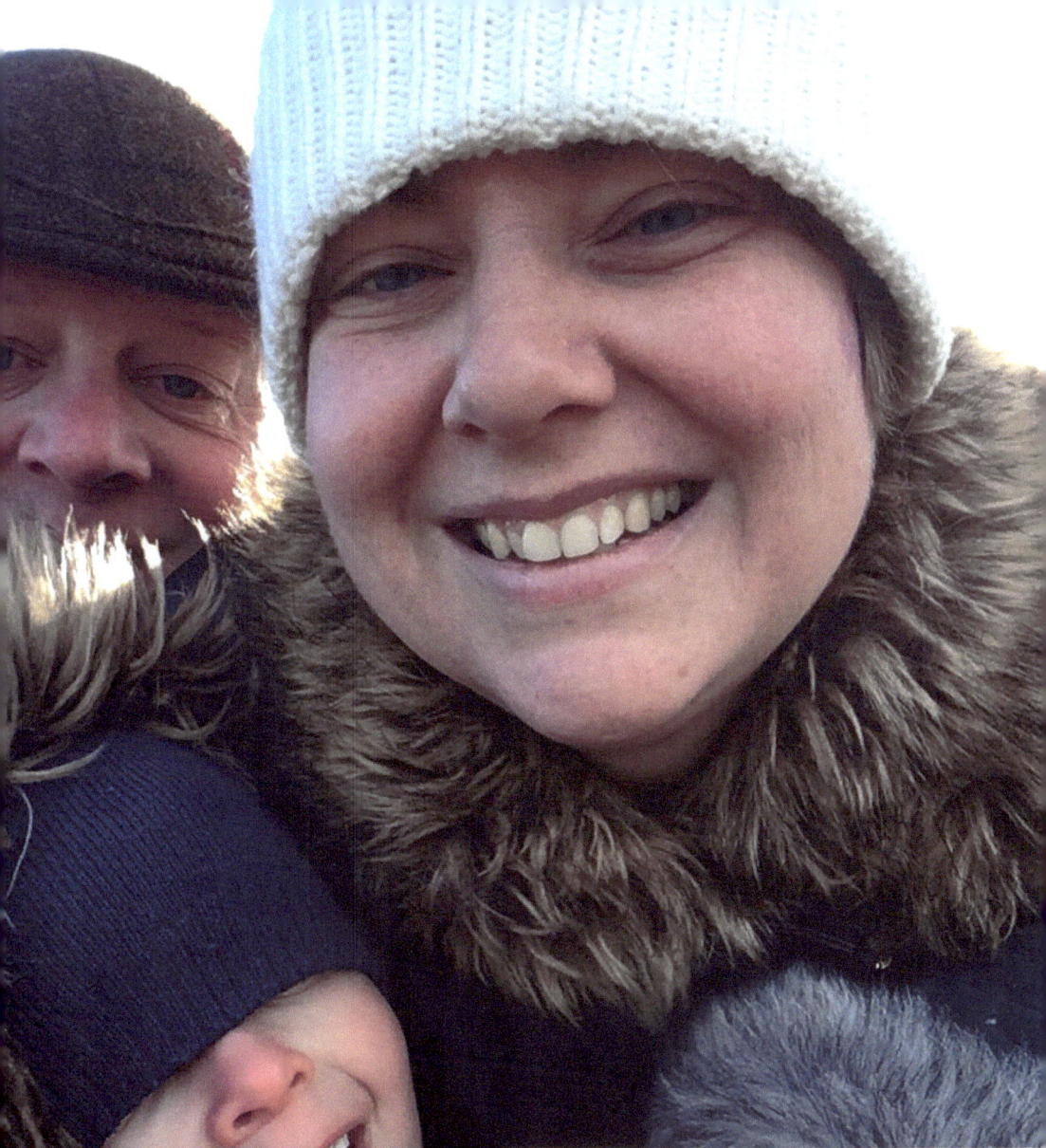

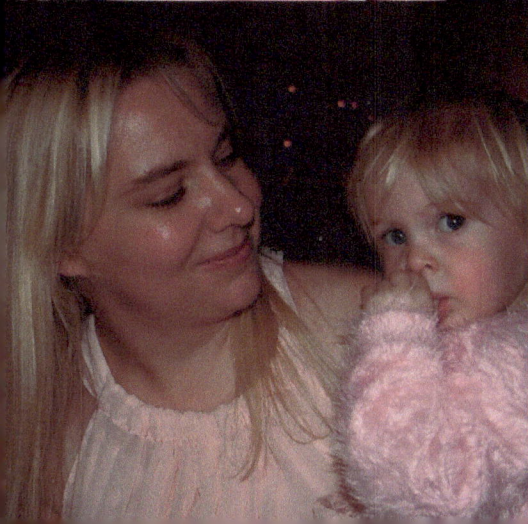

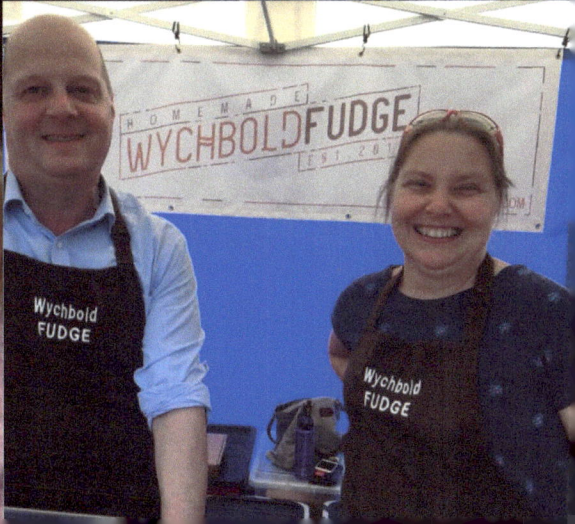

Justin Bowen is with **Helga Peeters**
12th August 2019 at 06:25

Good morning everyone

We now have the date for Helga's funeral. It will take place on Thursday 22nd August at 11.00am at St Mary De Wyche Church, Wychbold. It is open to everyone and a speaker system will relay the service to those who are outside the church.

We are asking people not to wear black, so please come dressed as brightly as you feel comfortable. We want a sea of colour.

We are also asking people not to send flowers. Instead we will be taking donations for Macmillan Cancer Support on the day. If people wish to have a single flower to throw on Helga's coffin as it passes or when it is placed in the ground that is fine.

Again I want to thank everyone for your love and support for the children and me.

You are all amazing.

❤️

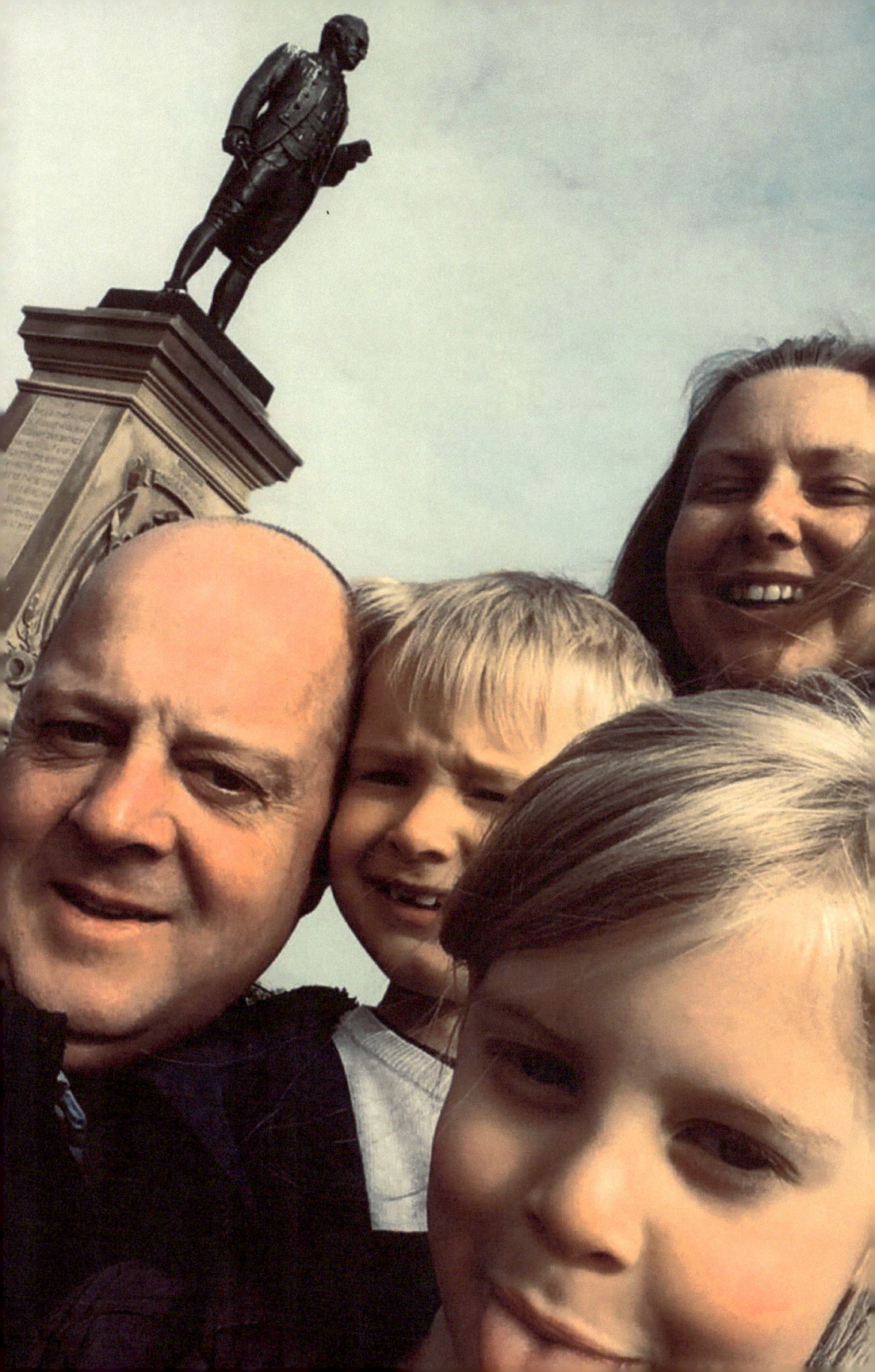

Justin Bowen is with **Helga Peeters**
22nd Aug 2019 at 07:57

Just over 12 years ago at our wedding, mine and Helga's first dance was to 'Dancing in the Moonlight' by Toploader. Today we'll have our last dance, for now. I'm no better at dancing now than I was then, so have no idea how it will go today. What I do know is that the children and I wouldn't have got through the last 3 weeks without you all. Thank you and see you later.

❤️

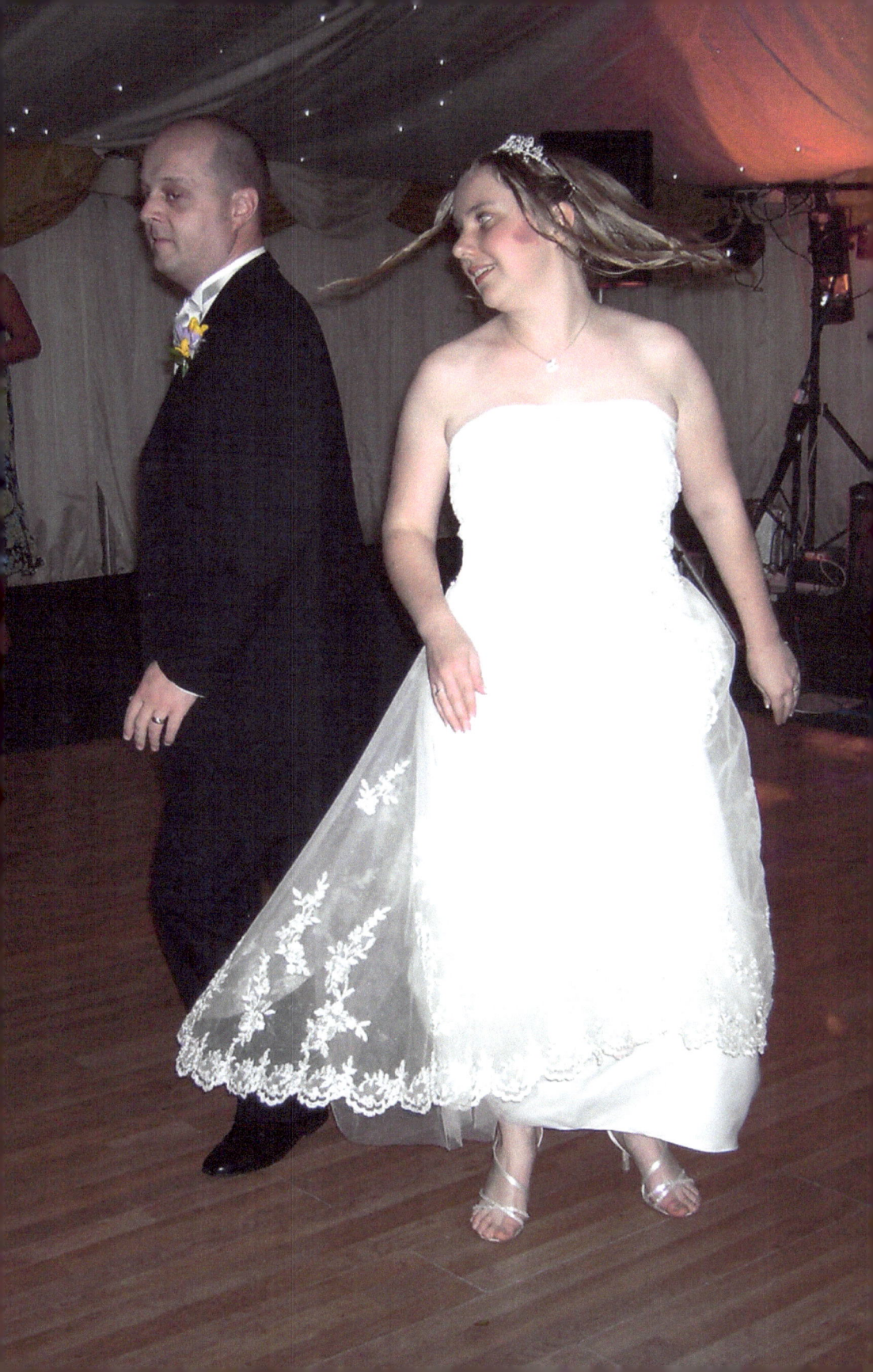

Justin Bowen is with **Helga Peeters**
23rd Aug 2019 at 08:05

Thank you to everyone who came yesterday. Your colours were wonderful and meant that when the children and I looked up from Helga's graveside we saw a rainbow. As Bren looked around he just said "Look at all these people Dad" It meant everything.

I'll be keeping Helga's Facebook page open, so if you ever feel like posting something on there you can. A thought, a memory, a moment.

Love to you all

❤️

PAGE 4   www.bromsgrovestandard.co.uk   The Standard, Friday August 30, 2019

Packed service remembers an inspirational, optimistic woman

by Tristan Harris
tristan.harris@bullivantmedia.com

MORE than 200 people packed into St Mary de Wyche Church last Thursday to pay tribute and bid a fond farewell to popular Wychbold Fudge co-founder Helga Peeters.

The striking blue summer sky coffin, reflecting Helga's ever-optimistic character, was led into the church to a poignant cover version of The Beatles' Golden Slumbers as the ceremony.

The service was led by Minister Angela Kovacevic and included words from Helga's family in Belgium which cited her as being 'determined from a very young age'.

She met Justin, her 'knight in shining armour', playing online game The Dark Age of Camelot and 'followed her heart to England'.

Friends' described her a 'truly inspirational person' who had a massive smile which radiated from her heart and left an impression on everyone she met.

She was always positive even when she was diagnosed with her illness, saying: "It is what it is" and "It's the way the cookie crumbles."

Helga was a wonderful mum who was so proud of her children and loved bringing people together, the congregation heard

She started numerous networking groups and would always organise social get-togethers which inevitably involved gin, prosecco, popcorn and, of course, fudge.

She was 'feisty, lively and full of fun', always the first on the dancefloor with her friends not being able to get her off it during 1980s and 90s themed nights.

Helga was easy-going, always organ-

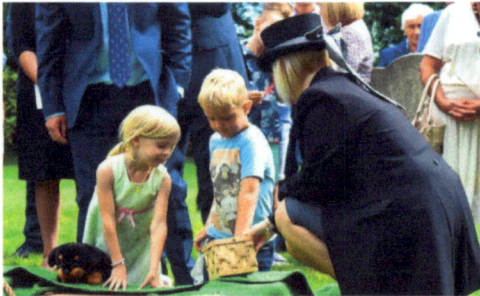

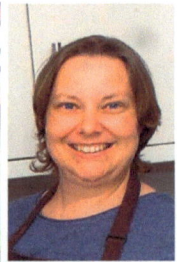

ised, a capable problem-solver and a true leader, added the friends' tribute.

When she was diagnosed she was always there for the other women in the cancer support group she joined.

She 'looked stunning' when she took to the catwalk in the group's charity fashion show that she encouraged others to join her in doing.

"Heaven has got its ultimate angel."

Another friend said: "We should not mourn that Helga's life was short but celebrate that we were part of her short life."

Moving words from son Brennan which were read out, remembering mummy as a very kind lady who was both 'fun and funny' and always offered 'warm cuddles'.

And husband Justin said Helga

brought people together because she wanted to be belong to a community which helped each other and one she felt proud to be part of.

Prayers were said by Rev Canon Wyn Beynon and hymns included Amazing Grace and Lord of the Dance.

The last song before the committal - Toploader's Dancing in the Moonlight - led to giggles throughout the church as

soon as the first notes came in.

After the coffin was lowered into the grave, friends and family members placed flowers on it and Brennan and Seren released two balloons - one red and one pink.

A collection on the day raised £1,275 for Macmillan Cancer Support and family and friends gathered in Wychbold Social Club afterwards.

Helga was remembered fondly after the service. Picture by Sarah Rooney. s

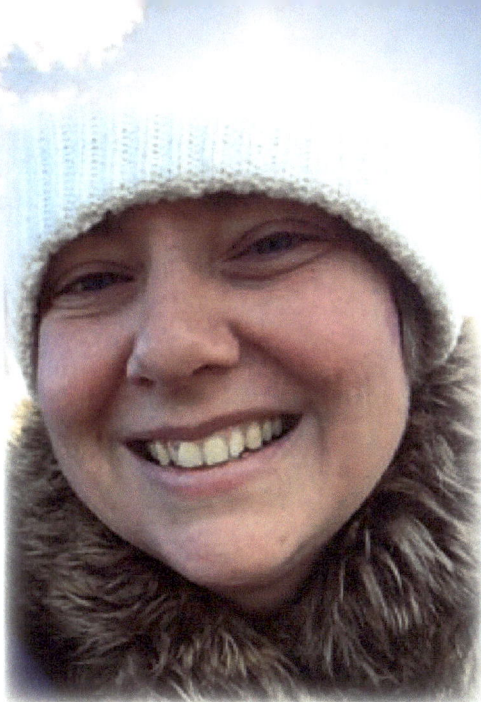

A Service of Celebration for the Life of

HELGA NOEL ANNA PEETERS

7th October 1982 - 5th August 2019

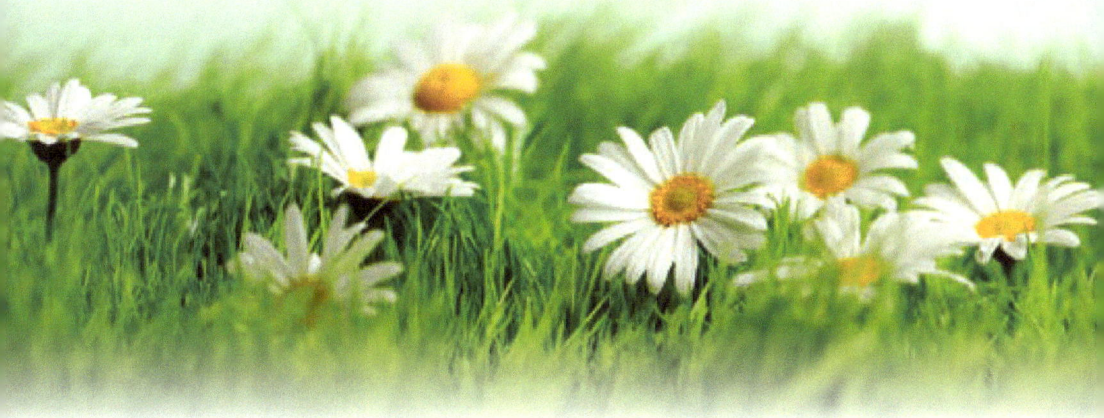

St Mary de Wyche Church, Wychbold

Thursday 22nd August 2019 at 11.00 am

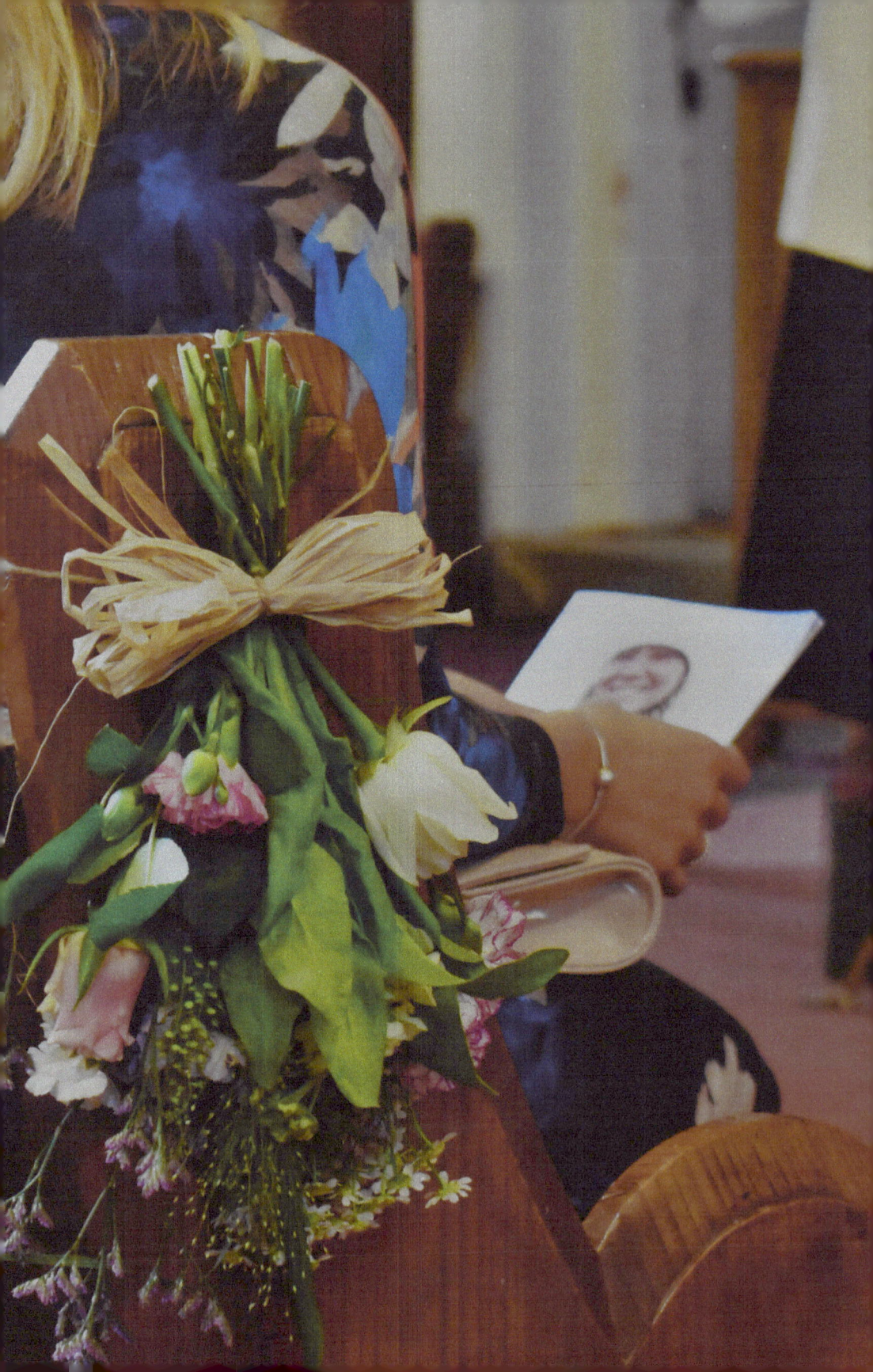

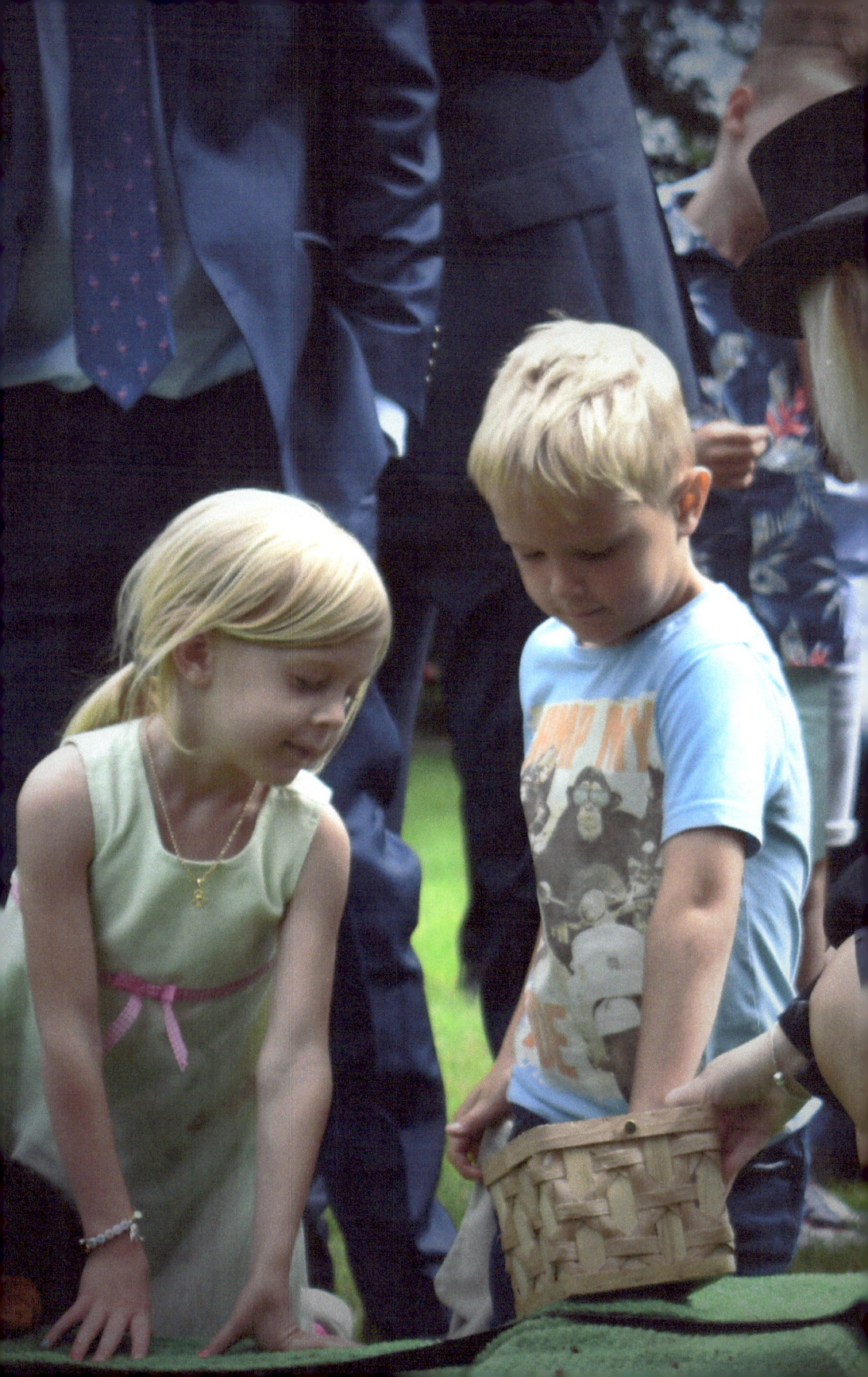

One Year On...

Justin Bowen
5th Aug 2020

It's a year today since Helga died. Thank you for the kind messages - it means a lot to know there will be many people thinking of her today.

A year on I thought I'd say a little of what it's been like. I won't be offended if you scroll on past at this point!

Much of it will be familiar to anyone who's lost someone. Maybe it will be useful to someone.

When your wife dies young and you have children to raise there are basically 3 lots of grief to bear.

Firstly, you grieve for your own loss – the life that you had that will be no more, the future that you imagined that will never be, how you & your family's life is now all on you. Secondly, you grieve for your wife's loss – for the things she'll never do, the places she'll never see, how she'll not see your children growing up, getting married, having your grandchildren. The life she's lost. Thirdly, you grieve for your children's loss – the time with their mum they'll not have, the cuddles they'll miss, the wisdom they'll not receive, the way everything will be different to how it was going to be.

Now thankfully this grief, it isn't constant. It comes in waves. Big waves, turbulent waves, crashing over you. And in those moments that a huge breaker is bearing down, you can do one of 2 things.

Either you let it smash you against the rocks, breaking you into pieces, or you become the rock – digging deep, letting each wave break on you, weathering the storm and being weathered by it, until it passes.

Then, when the calm settles and the sun comes out, you get to look around and see that you're still there, that there is so much to appreciate and enjoy and that your children still need you. And that's your motivation when the next one hits.

So, at first, after losing your companion, your best friend, your confidant, the person you love the most, those waves come one after the other after the other.

Relentless, with never a moment between. Each one threatening to wash you away. But gradually, as time goes on and you weather each storm, gaps start to appear.

There is a lull between each one, and that lull grows imperceptibly longer each time. Moments to breathe, to gather yourself, to start to think about what next.

Now don't get me wrong – the waves can still be big. They can catch you unaware and stop you in your tracks. But the weathering of them becomes more familiar and you gain strength from that. You realise you're doing it; you're getting through.

A year on and today, at some point, there will likely be a storm. But it will pass and the children and I will carry on with our new life. I made a promise to Helga on the day she died that we would have a good life. I said it so that Helga knew it was safe for her to go. I also said it because it's true. I miss her loads, but we're doing ok.

Thanks for all your love and support.

Justin

❤️

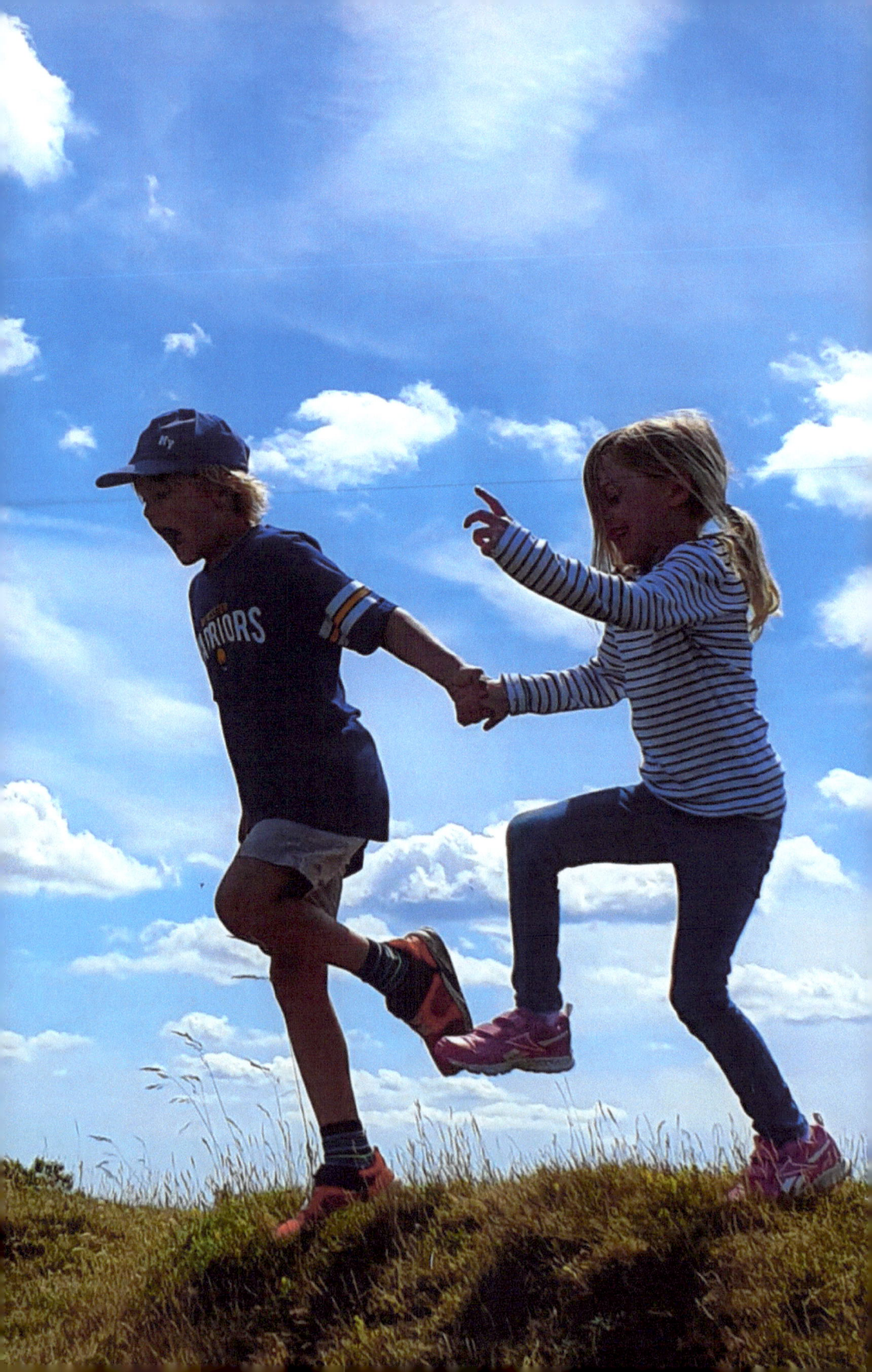

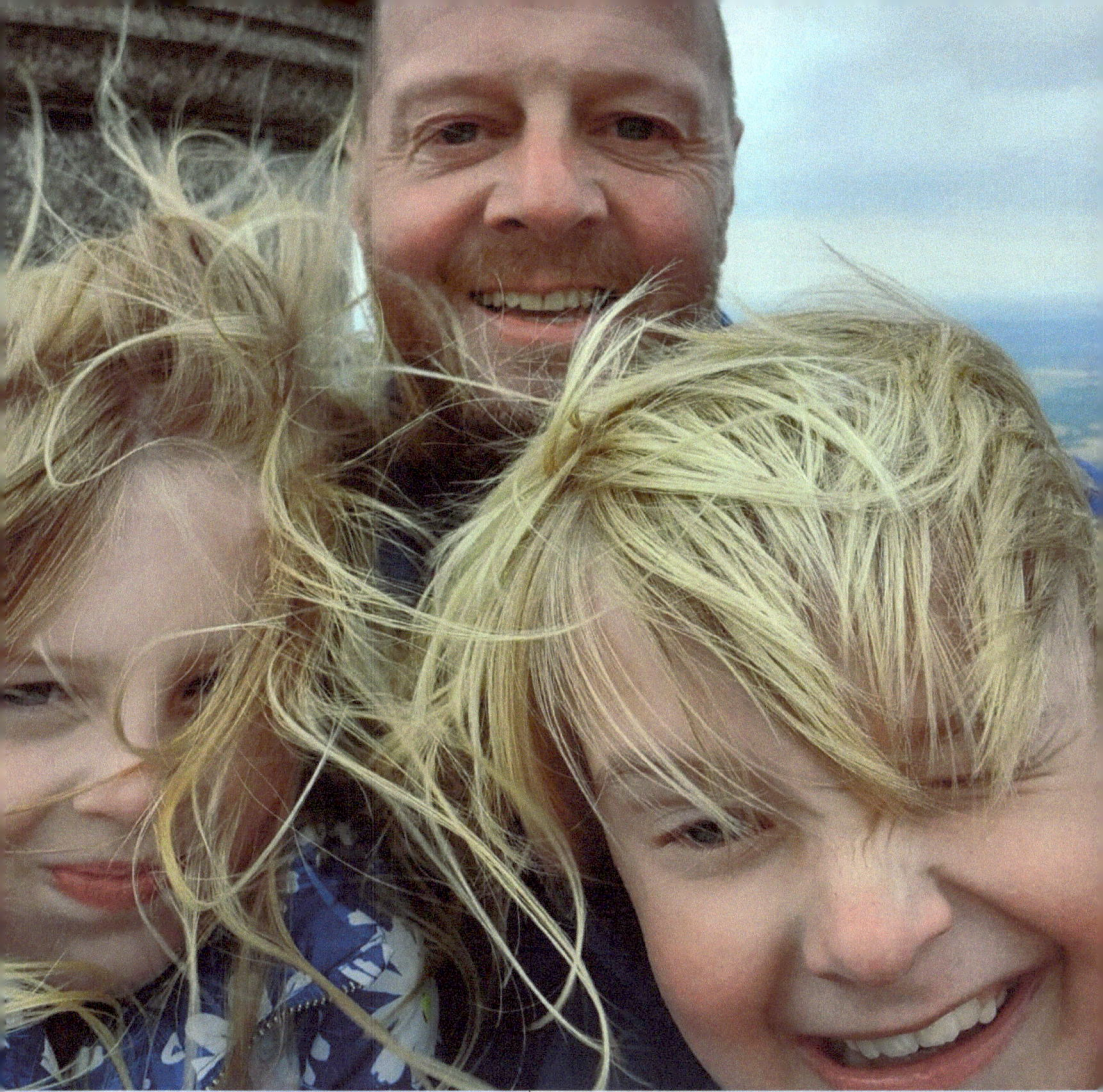

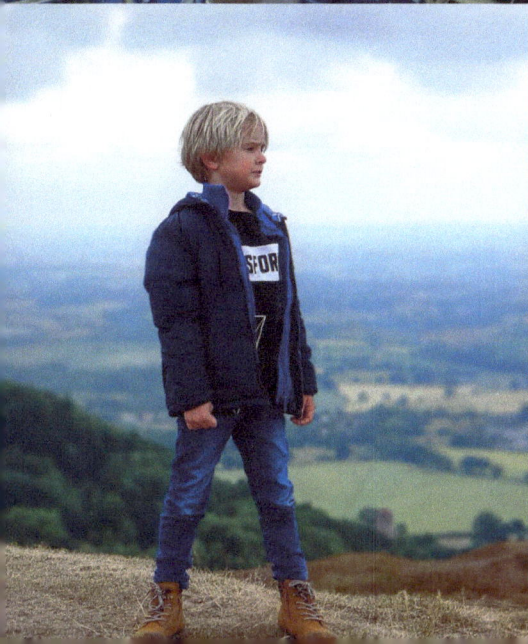

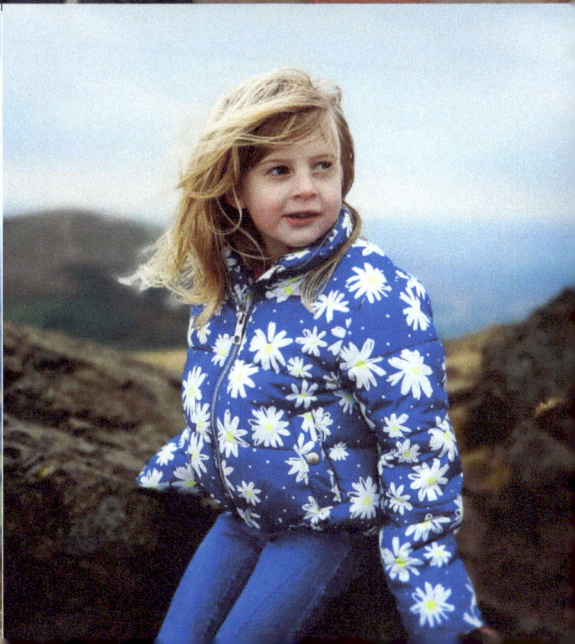